Navigating Life with Parkinson Disease

Navigating Life with Parkinson Disease

Sotirios A. Parashos, MD, PhD

Minneapolis Clinic of Neurology;
Struthers Parkinson's Center
Park Nicollet Methodist Hospital
Golden Valley, MN; and
Department of Neurology
University of Minnesota
Minneapolis, MN

Rose L. Wichmann, PT

Struthers Parkinson's Center
Park Nicollet Methodist Hospital
Golden Valley, MN; and
Allied Team Training Program
National Parkinson Foundation

Todd Melby

Minneapolis, MN

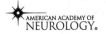

AMERICAN ACADEMY OF
NEUROLOGY®

OXFORD
UNIVERSITY PRESS

Oxford University Press is a department of the University of Oxford.
It furthers the University's objective of excellence in research, scholarship, and education by publishing
worldwide.

Oxford   New York

Auckland   Cape Town   Dar es Salaam   Hong Kong   Karachi
Kuala Lumpur   Madrid   Melbourne   Mexico City   Nairobi
New Delhi   Shanghai   Taipei   Toronto

With offices in

Argentina   Austria   Brazil   Chile   Czech Republic   France   Greece
Guatemala   Hungary   Italy   Japan   Poland   Portugal   Singapore
South Korea   Switzerland   Thailand   Turkey   Ukraine   Vietnam

Oxford is a registered trade mark of Oxford University Press in the UK
and certain other countries.

Published in the United States of America by
Oxford University Press
198 Madison Avenue, New York, NY 10016

First issued as an Oxford University Press paperback, 2013

Library of Congress Cataloging-in-Publication Data
Parashos, Sotirios A.
Navigating life with Parkinson disease / Sotirios A. Parashos,
Rose L. Wichmann, Todd Melby.
p. cm.
Includes index.
ISBN 978–0–19–989778–0 (pbk)
1. Parkinson's disease—Patients.   2. Parkinson's disease—
Patients—Rehabilitation.   3. Self-care, Health.   I. Wichmann, Rose L.
II. Melby, Todd.   III. Title.
RC382.P3497 2013
616.8′33—dc23
2012011187

This material is not intended to be, and should not be considered, a substitute for medical or other
professional advice. Treatment for the conditions described in this material is highly dependent on the
individual circumstances. And, while this material is designed to offer accurate information with respect
to the subject matter covered and to be current as of the time it was written, research and knowledge
about medical and health issues is constantly evolving and dose schedules for medications are being
revised continually, with new side effects recognized and accounted for regularly. Readers must therefore
always check the product information and clinical procedures with the most up-to-date published product
information and data sheets provided by the manufacturers and the most recent codes of conduct and
safety regulation. The publisher and the authors make no representations or warranties to readers,
express or implied, as to the accuracy or completeness of this material. Without limiting the foregoing, the
publisher and the authors make no representations or warranties as to the accuracy or efficacy of the drug
dosages mentioned in the material. The authors and the publisher do not accept, and expressly disclaim,
any responsibility for any liability, loss or risk that may be claimed or incurred as a consequence of the use
and/or application of any of the contents of this material.

Disclosure statements for potential conflicts of interest provided by the authors are available
upon request from the American Academy of Neurology, 201 Chicago Avenue, Minneapolis,
MN 55415; Attn: *Neurology Now Books*.

3 5 7 9 8 6 4
Printed in the United States of America on acid-free paper

CONTENTS

14. Planning For Your Future: Managing Your Personal Affairs | 235

Murray Sagsveen, JD, and Laurie Hanson, JD

ABOUT THE AAN'S *NEUROLOGY NOW*™ BOOK SERIES

Here is a question for you:

If you know more about your neurologic condition, will you do better than if you know less?

Well, it's not simply optimism but hard data that show that individuals who are more knowledgeable about their medical conditions *do have better outcomes.* So learning about your neurologic condition plays an important role in doing the very best you can. The main purpose of both the American Academy of Neurology's (AAN's) *Neurology Now*™ book series and *Neurology Now* magazine is to focus on the needs of people with neurologic disorders. Our goal is to view neurologic issues through the eyes of people with neurologic problems, in order to understand and respond to their practical day-to-day needs.

So, you are probably saying, *"Of course, knowledge is a good thing, but how can it change the course of my disease?"* Well, health care is really a two-way street. You need to find a knowledgeable and trusted neurologist; however, no physician can overcome the obstacle of working with inaccurate or incomplete information. Your physician is working to navigate the clues you provide in your own words combined with the clues from their neurologic examination, in order to arrive at an accurate diagnosis and respond to your individual needs. Many types of important clues exist, such as your description of your symptoms or your ability to identify how your neurologic condition affects your daily activities. Poor patient-physician communication inevitably results in less-than-ideal outcomes. This problem is well described by the old adage, "garbage in, garbage out." The better you pin down and communicate your main problem(s), the more likely you are to walk out of your doctor's office with the plan that is right for you. Your neurologist is the expert in your disorder, but you and your family are the experts in "you." Physician decision making is not a "one shoe fits all" enterprise, yet when accurate, individualized information is lacking, that's what it becomes.

Whether you are startled by hearing a new diagnosis or you come to this knowledge gradually, learning that you have a neurologic problem is jarring. Many neurologic disorders are chronic; you aren't simply adjusting to something new—you will need to deal with this disorder for the foreseeable future. In certain ways, life has changed. Now, there are two crucial "next steps": the first is finding good neurologic care for your problem, and the second is successfully adjusting to living with your condition. This second step depends on attaining knowledge of your condition, learning new skills to manage the condition, and finding the flexibility and resourcefulness to restore your quality of life. When successful, you regain your equilibrium and restore a sense of confidence and control that is the cornerstone of well-being.

When healthy adjustment does not occur following a new diagnosis, a sense of feeling out of control and overwhelmed often persists, and no doctor's prescription will adequately respond to this problem. Individuals who acquire good self-management skills are often able to recognize and understand new symptoms and take appropriate action. Conversely, those who are lacking in confidence may respond to the same symptom with a growing sense of anxiety and urgency. In the first case, "watchful waiting" or a call to the physician may result in resolution of the problem. In the second case, the uncertainty and anxiety often lead to multiple physician consultations, unnecessary new prescriptions, social withdrawal, or unwarranted hospitalization. Outcomes can be dramatically different depending on knowledge and preparedness.

Managing a neurologic disorder is new territory, and you should not be surprised that you need to be equipped with new information and a new skill set to effectively manage your condition. You will need to learn new words that describe both your symptoms and their treatment to communicate effectively with the members of your medical team. You will also need to learn how to gather accurate information about your condition when you need it and to avoid misinformation. Although all of your physicians document your progress in their medical records, keeping a personal journal about your neurologic condition will help you summarize and track all your medical information in one place. When you bring this journal with you as you go to see your physician, you will be able to provide more accurate information about your history and previous treatment. Your active and informed involvement in your care and decision making results in a better quality of care and better outcomes.

Your neurologic condition is likely to pose new challenges in daily activities, including interactions in your family, your workplace, and your social and recreational activities. How can you best manage your symptoms or your medication dosing schedule in the context of your normal activities? When should you disclose your diagnosis to others? *Neurology Now* Books provide you with the background you need, including the experiences of others who have faced similar problems, to guide you through this unfamiliar terrain. Our goal is to give you the resources you need to "take your doctor with you" when you confront these new challenges. We are committed to answering the questions and concerns of individuals living with neurologic disorders and their families in each volume of the *Neurology Now* book series. We want you to be as prepared and confident as possible to participate with your doctors in your medical care. Much care is taken to develop each book with you in mind. A special authorship model takes a multidisciplinary team approach to put together the most up-to-date, informative, and useful answers to the questions that most concern you—whether you find yourself in the unexpected role of patient or caregiver. Each authorship team includes neurologists with special expertise along with a diversity of other contributors with special knowledge of the particular neurologic disorder. Depending on the specific condition, this includes rehabilitation specialists, nurses, social workers, and people or family members with important shared experiences. Professional writers work to ensure that we avoid "doctor talk," and easy-to-understand definitions of new terms appear on the page when a new word is introduced. Real-life experiences of patients and families are found throughout the text to illustrate important points. And feedback based on correspondence from *Neurology Now* magazine readers informs topics for new books and is integral to our quality improvement. These new features will be found in all books in the *Neurology Now* book series so that you can expect the same quality and patient-centered approach in every volume.

I hope that you have arrived at a new understanding of why "knowledge is empowering" when it comes to your medical care and that *Neurology Now* Books will serve as an important foundation for the new skills you need to be effective in managing a neurologic condition.

Lisa M. Shulman, MD
Editor-In-Chief, *Neurology Now* Book Series
and Professor of Neurology
University of Maryland School of Medicine

FOREWORD

As mortals with finite life spans, we unconsciously recognize that middle age and beyond will be associated with medical conditions. However, when confronted with an age-related neurologic "disease" we tend to panic. This is especially true with Parkinson's disease, which has gained much publicity in recent years. Famous athletes have become disabled with this condition, and relatives or friends may be in nursing homes with Parkinson's disease.

Knowledge about their condition is crucial to people with any major disorder, and certainly this is true for Parkinson's disease. The early panic and initial despair at the diagnosis can be tempered by knowledge. Parkinson's disease compromises lives, but it is treatable. With optimal treatment, people with Parkinson's disease can often lead quite normal lives for many, many years. Obviously, this varies among individuals, but the diagnosis should not be regarded as a death sentence. For example, in Olmsted County, Minnesota (where I live), people with Parkinson's disease live to ages within three years of the life spans that would be predicted without the disease.

The primary author of this book, Dr. Sotirios Parashos, and the other contributors are to be congratulated for writing this comprehensive text for people with Parkinson's disease and their families.

It was written under the auspices of the American Academy of Neurology, a physician organization that demands fair and balanced works. They have addressed all the fundamental issues that confront individuals with Parkinson's disease, defining terms and providing a balanced discussion. In the present era of electronic media and the Internet, we are constantly confronted with medical "facts." Moreover, it is easy to use a search engine to find information about virtually anything, including Parkinson's disease. Of course, the problem with the lay press is that the medical information is not always vetted. The Internet dogmatically provides all sorts of information, but how much of it is true? Consequently, an unbiased and comprehensive book for people with Parkinson's disease is crucial, and this text provides a myriad of information that will serve the Parkinson's disease community well.

As you read this book, be reassured by the fact that Parkinson's disease is treatable; the goal for clinicians such as me is to keep people in the mainstreams of their lives. As you will read, exercise and activity are very important for people with Parkinson's disease, and optimum medical treatment is therefore crucial to allow such exercise. Philosophies about Parkinson's disease treatment vary among clinicians. This is evident if you use the U.S. National Library of Medicine search engine, PubMed; enter the search term "Parkinson's disease treatment," and approximately 34,000 published articles surface. If you scan some of the more-recent entries, you will realize that treatment approaches are quite varied. The authors of this book needed to be cognizant of those differing approaches while avoiding legitimization of marginal therapies. Thus the treatment chapters take a very comprehensive view of what is available and how clinicians of disparate therapeutic philosophies might select specific drugs or therapies. This background will be invaluable for patients when interacting with their personal clinicians and also when reading Internet entries.

Family and caregivers are important members of the Parkinson's disease team. Knowledge about this condition will help them understand the lifestyle compromises that surface to variable extents over the course of this disorder. As we age, we all will need family and caregivers, and for those with Parkinson's disease this is especially true. They also will appreciate this book.

J. Eric Ahlskog, PhD, MD
Consultant in Neurology, Mayo Clinic, Rochester, MN
Professor of Neurology, Mayo Medical School

Author of another Oxford University Press book for those with Parkinson's disease: *The Parkinson's Disease Treatment Book: Partnering with Your Doctor to Get the Most from Your Medications*

PREFACE

In an era where information on just about everything that has to do with health and illness is for many people only a few keystrokes away, it is only natural to ask, "Why one more book about Parkinson disease?"

The reasons for this undertaking are multiple but have a lot to do precisely with the fact that information about Parkinson disease is abundant and accessible. For people recently diagnosed with the disease and their loved ones it quickly becomes a daunting task just to navigate through all this information, not to mention to be able to sort out the reliable from the not-so-reliable sources. For people in the more-advanced stages of the disease who seek specific answers to their specific problems, there can very easily be too much information. It is great news that research has expanded our understanding of Parkinson disease in the last decade, but it has also created a maze of possibilities and directions that is very hard to follow, quite often even for the scientists and physicians who have dedicated their lives in the fight to conquer this disease.

Considering the "lay of the land," it would be irrational to even suggest that the book in your hands constitutes a comprehensive review of the disease. It can, however, be a good compass both to the uninitiated and to the "old hands." The text will take you through the basics of Parkinson's, the theories about its causes, the symptoms of its various stages, and the available treatments, including medications, therapies, and brain surgery. More importantly, whole chapters are dedicated to day-to-day management of the disease symptoms, strategies to improve function and ameliorate quality of life, and even legal and financial advice. A number of resources are cited so that the interested reader can seek further information through reliable, authoritative Web sites. The information presented in this book is accompanied by illustrative examples and true stories relating experiences of persons with Parkinson's and their care partners. We have asked Parkinson's experts to give us their "two cents" on some "hot topics," and these vignettes are easily identifiable and set apart from the main text for easy access and reference. For more practical items, we adopted a Q&A format for easy assimilation of the information.

This book was truly a group effort. We would like to thank our expert panel for their knowledgeable insights and the persons with Parkinson's and their care partners who were very kind to share their experiences for this book. We would like to thank Dr. Brent Clark of the University of Minnesota for providing us with photographs of the Lewy body and the substantia nigra. We also thank Rick Vandendolder, OTR, of the Struthers Parkinson's Center for his help with photographing adaptive equipment for people with Parkinson's. Dr. Lisa Shulman, series editor, and Ms. Andrea Weiss of the Neurology Now series were very supportive throughout this effort. Craig Panner of Oxford University Press can be credited for making sure the book made sense as a whole and has been particularly helpful, patient, and accommodating throughout the process of publishing the book.

Last but not least, we would like to thank the Parkinson disease community, a very proactive group of people, who make our efforts so much easier with their support and dedication to our common goal.

Navigating Life with Parkinson Disease

Chapter 1

Introduction

Terry plays basketball on weekends. For a few weeks, he had noticed an occasional slight tremor in his right hand, which he thought was strange, because he didn't remember banging it during a game. Then he noticed that sometimes the tiny shaking in his hand occurred when he walked. And sometimes it happened when he wasn't doing anything—he'd just be standing, his arm at his side, and the trembling, ever so mild, would begin. Terry, a healthy man in his mid-40s, didn't give any of this much thought. He was too busy with his life: during the day, he had a challenging job as an executive at a successful advertising agency, and at home, he enjoyed relaxing with his wife. One morning, he got out of bed to go to the bathroom and his wife saw his right hand shaking. It wasn't pronounced, but it was a definite shake. She talked to Terry about it, and he told her about other times it had happened. They decided he should go see a doctor. After an examination, Terry's doctor told him he had Parkinson disease (Parkinson's for short).

Like Terry, about 1.5 million Americans are living with Parkinson disease. Older people are more likely to get Parkinson disease than younger people: the average age of diagnosis is 67 years old. But about 15 percent of people with Parkinson's begin showing symptoms before the age of 50, and the disease can be seen in much younger people. About two out of every 100 people over the age of 70 are living with Parkinson disease. The disease affects both men and women and people of all ethnic groups.

Parkinson disease is named for James Parkinson, a London physician who wrote the book *An Essay on the Shaking Palsy* (see Figure 1–1) about the illness in 1817. Originally called "shaking palsy" or "paralysis agitans," it was later renamed Parkinson disease by Charcot, a famous French neurologist of the 19th century. In his book, Parkinson defined the condition he had observed in patients this way: "Involuntary tremulous motion, with lessened muscular power, in parts not in action and even when supported; with a propensity to bend the trunk forwards, and to pass from a walking to a running pace: the senses and intellects being uninjured." Through the years, we have come to recognize

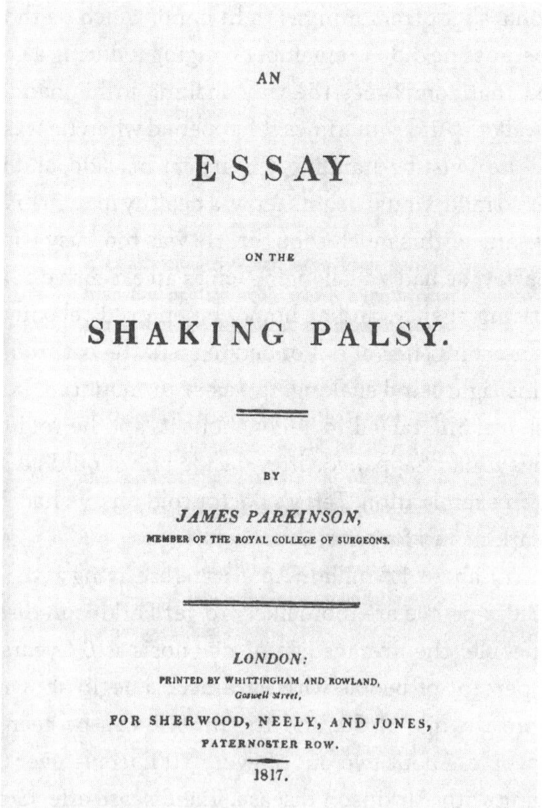

AN

ESSAY

ON THE

SHAKING PALSY.

BY

JAMES PARKINSON,
MEMBER OF THE ROYAL COLLEGE OF SURGEONS.

LONDON:
PRINTED BY WHITTINGHAM AND ROWLAND,
Goswell Street,

FOR SHERWOOD, NEELY, AND JONES,
PATERNOSTER ROW.

1817.

FIGURE 1-1 Frontispiece of James Parkinson's *Essay on the Shaking Palsy.*

that the main target of Parkinson disease is in the brain. Normally, a small cluster of nerve cells (or **neurons**) called the **substantia nigra**, which is located in the brainstem, produces **dopamine**, a chemical that is essential to smooth movement. The disease is a neurodegenerative disorder. The word **neurodegenerative** indicates a premature death of neurons. In Parkinson disease, the dopamine-producing (or **dopaminergic**) neurons of the substantia nigra die prematurely. For this reason, the brains of people with Parkinson's are deficient in dopamine, and the result is loss of smooth, full-range motion.

The exact cause of Parkinson disease is unknown: despite years of research, we still don't understand what kills these dopaminergic neurons. Some researchers have identified certain environmental factors that may increase one's chances of developing the disease. An example of such environmental influences is exposure to pesticides and other chemicals that are common on farms and ranches: North Dakota (one of the most rural areas in the United States) has the highest rate of Parkinson disease in the nation. In some people, the cause of Parkinson disease can be found in their genes.

Early signs of Parkinson disease include smaller handwriting, a soft voice, reduced facial expression, slowness of movement, tremor, and changes in walking (shuffling) and posture (stooping). Not all Parkinson's patients have all of these symptoms. To be diagnosed with Parkinson disease, a person needs to exhibit at least two of the four "cardinal" symptoms, which are tremor, bradykinesia (slowed movement), rigidity, and postural instability. Because the diagnosis is difficult to make, some specialists have proposed that Parkinson disease cannot be diagnosed unless bradykinesia is one of the two symptoms.

> Parkinson disease happens because of the premature death of **dopamine**-producing nerve cells in the **substantia nigra**. The exact cause of the disease is unknown.

Parkinson's is a remarkably individualized disease. Nearly every person's story is different. One person may experience tremor at the early stages of the disease; another person may experience tremor at a later stage of the disease or even not at all; in yet others, new symptoms may replace tremor as the disease progresses. One of the things that are true for all Parkinson's patients is that the disease progresses over time. In the beginning, a person may have only a few symptoms, but new symptoms will usually develop later on. The dopamine-producing neurons will continue to die, the amount of dopamine in the brain will continue to decline, and a person's symptoms will get worse. Depending on a wide variety of factors—including age, severity of the illness, medication, and exercise—some people may experience more intrusive, sometimes even disabling, symptoms over years or decades. Others may have a very slow progression of the symptoms and can live very productive lives without any significant impairment.

The "Cardinal Symptoms" of Parkinson Disease Explained

- **Tremor**: Shaking of a hand, arm, foot, leg, chin, or lips. In Parkinson disease this happens while the limb is at rest, but sometimes it happens also with movement.
- **Bradykinesia**: Unusually slow movement of the limbs or the entire body.
- **Rigidity**: Stiffness of the muscles in the hand, arm, foot, leg, or the trunk and neck.
- **Postural Instability**: Wobbly or unbalanced standing or walking.

Although physical symptoms are the first indications of the disease, many Parkinson's patients also experience behavioral changes such as fatigue, apathy, depression, anxiety, and sleep problems.

These behavioral symptoms will be explored in more detail in Chapter 4.

> **Progression** of Parkinson disease varies from person to person, but it may be slow and in some cases may never lead to significant impairment.

Medication can be very effective in treating the symptoms of Parkinson disease. There are medications that encourage the production of dopamine in the brain or actually supply the brain with a substitute for dopamine. Other medications help the brain make better use of its remaining dopamine-producing capacity. Yet other medications may suppress naturally occurring chemicals that work against dopamine. All these medications help reduce shakiness, slowness, stiffness, and other symptoms in most patients.

> Many famous people found **inspiration and new meaning** in their lives after they were diagnosed with Parkinson disease.

In addition to medication, certain types of therapies can also help alleviate parkinsonian symptoms. Physical, occupational, and speech therapies may lead to surprising improvement of the physical symptoms, though brain surgery may be necessary when symptom control becomes unpredictable. For many people, exercise also helps reduce the symptoms associated with the disease. We'll discuss these treatments later in the book (Chapters 8, 9, and 10).

You Are Not Alone

When Parkinson's patients get together and share their stories, they quickly learn about the variety of ways people are affected by the illness. Many people also benefit from telling others about their experience, hearing others' experiences, and learning ways to live with the disease.

Several famous Americans have been diagnosed with Parkinson disease, including boxer Muhammad Ali, former Attorney General Janet Reno, and the actor Michael J. Fox. These inspiring people have shown that it is possible to live a fulfilling life with Parkinson disease. It may not be the life Ali, Reno, or Fox thought they were going to live when they imagined their lives decades ago, but it can be a rewarding one.

Imagine being the world's greatest boxer, at the height of one's powers, dancing around the ring with style, grace, and speed. Imagine being a thoughtful attorney who enjoys hiking in parks in your spare time. Imagine being one of the nation's best-known actors, famous in movies and television, handsome, cool, and in control. Ali, Reno, and Fox didn't imagine their lives would be affected by Parkinson disease, yet they have been. All three are living with the disease in their own individual ways, because Parkinson's has affected their movements, their physical abilities, in individualized ways. But each has continued to live a very productive life.

Muhammad Ali lit the torch at the 1996 Olympics in Atlanta, his hands shaking as he did so, and continues to be a very effective advocate for the Parkinson Disease community. Reno, an avid hiker, switched to canoeing after Parkinson's made it too difficult to hike. But she remained active. Meanwhile, Michael J. Fox created a foundation that supports Parkinson's research and has continued acting, appearing on TV shows such as *Scrubs*, *Boston Legal*, and *Rescue Me*.

About This Book and How to Use It

In this book, we will focus on Parkinson disease itself, clarify some misunderstandings, describe the symptoms that may occur in different stages of the disease, explore possible causes, describe how the disease is diagnosed, and discuss what can be done to treat the symptoms. We'll also discuss complications of the various treatments, suggest steps you can take to improve your prognosis, write about ongoing research, explore new treatment options, and suggest ways for you to continue to live a productive and rewarding life.

It has been the experience of the authors of this book, but also of the many physicians and health care professionals who treat Parkinson disease, that one of the most important factors for successful disease management is informed patients (and care partners). In the modern approach to chronic disease management, the patient is placed at the center of the "team." In an analogy to government, the patient becomes the "president" and remains in charge of his or her care. The doctor acts as a "chief of staff," while other health care professionals become "cabinet members." This model calls for patient-centered, multidisciplinary, and interdisciplinary disease management.

Elements of Successful Disease Management
- Informed patient (and care partner or family)
- Multidisciplinary team of health care professionals
- Communication
- Respect for patient's priorities and wishes

"Patient-centered" means what was just described. "Multidisciplinary" means that health care professionals from many fields (such as physical, occupational, or speech therapists; nurses; psychologists; or exercise physiologists) may need to provide their expert assessments and specialized treatments at various stages of the disease. "Interdisciplinary" means that all these health care professionals, including the doctor, need to communicate, consult with each other, and act as a team, with the aim of addressing the patient's health care needs and concerns while also paying attention to his or her wishes and expectations.

> While knowing more about the disease is important, available information can be overwhelming. Make your **learning decisions**—that is, your decisions about what (and what not) to learn—based on your personal preferences and needs and understand that you may wish to learn smaller amounts of information at a time.

In the first few chapters of this book (2 through 6), we try to explain the nature of the disease in terms of its symptoms, possible underlying causes, the anatomical and chemical changes that occur in the nervous system of persons living with the disease, and the various challenges patients have to face as the disease progresses. We cannot stress enough, however, how different the disease is from individual to individual. Therefore, it should not be thought that everything in this book applies to everyone who lives with Parkinson's.

In the second part of the book (Chapters 7 through 10), we address ways to manage the symptoms of the disease, including medications, exercise, therapies, surgical treatments, and lifestyle changes that may help address the challenges of living with Parkinson's. This is followed by chapters (11 through 14) dedicated to the role of research, planning for the future, how the care partner or the patient's family can be part of the disease management strategy, and how to become involved in advocating for the Parkinson's community. Finally, we include a glossary of technical terms at the end of the book.

We thought that real people's stories could help others understand their own challenges better and help them develop their own strategies for dealing with the disease. Therefore, throughout the book we have included real-life stories. In most instances, names, story details, and circumstances have been altered to conceal the person's identity.

Sometimes people want straightforward answers to very specific, frequently asked questions. We have sprinkled such "pearls of wisdom" from experts in the field in the form of "Ask the Experts" text boxes for quick reference.

This book cannot be either very detailed or all-encompassing. It is meant to be used as a guide. The best adviser for an individual with Parkinson disease will be a doctor—the quarterback of her or his "team."

Chapter 2

What Is It? Why Me?

Count de Lordat was a "handsome, middle-sized, sanguine man, of cheerful disposition, and an active mind." Unfortunately, de Lordat began losing control of his voice and left arm. At first, his speech was merely "a small impediment in uttering some words," but several months later, he had "difficulty in speaking." His left arm "withered more and more," becoming weaker and weaker. That's how one patient is described in James Parkinson's book *An Essay on the Shaking Palsy*. Parkinson wasn't the first person to notice symptoms associated with "the shaking palsy." Ancient Chinese manuscripts and medieval texts described people having the characteristic symptoms of the disease, like tremors, slow movements, shuffling, and stooping. But it's quite possible that not many people had the condition in those days. Most people living with Parkinson disease are older than 60, and until the past century or so, people lived much shorter lives. Moreover, it was much easier to attribute Parkinson's symptoms to aging.

From a functional standpoint, Parkinson disease is considered a **hypokinetic** disorder. "Hypo" is a Greek term meaning "under," while "kinesis" means "motion." Being hypokinetic simply means that people with Parkinson disease lack range and speed of motion in their movements. To many readers, this might not seem correct. After all, the symptom that most people associate with Parkinson's is tremor, which is an excess of motion. Although tremor is the most visible symptom of the disease, the central symptom of Parkinson's is a slowing of movements and a stiffening of the muscles like that seen in the case of Count de Lordat.

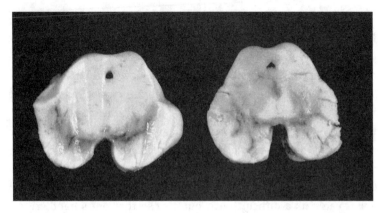

FIGURE 2-1 Substantia nigra from a normal brain (left) and that of a Parkinson's patient (right).

What Is It?

Parkinson disease is a **neurodegenerative** disorder. In neurodegenerative diseases neurons (nerve cells) die sooner than normal, both inside and outside the brain;most damage, however, occurs inside the brain. Humans are born with a specific number of neurons. As we age, many of these cells die a "natural" death. However, we are born with hundreds of billions of neurons in our brains, and under normal conditions we have plenty of "extra" nerve cells to keep the body and mind working well despite the losses. Unlike other cells, nerve cells do not reproduce to generate new nerve cells when something goes wrong. If a person loses part of the liver, the remaining liver cells will divide and multiply to produce new liver cells to replace some of the liver tissue that was lost. Another example is blood: blood cells are constantly produced by the bone marrow throughout our lives. However, when neurons die, the remaining ones can't multiply to produce new neurons. In neurodegenerative diseases certain types of neurons die at a much faster rate than normal "wear and tear" and are not replaced.

As discussed in Chapter 1, the neurons most affected in Parkinson disease are the dopaminergic neurons that live in a part of the brainstem called the substantia nigra—Latin for "black substance." The reason this part of the brain was called "black substance" is that it looks black in normal brains (as seen on the left in Figure 2–1). In Parkinson disease, however, the substantia nigra turns pale (as seen on the right in Figure 2–1). The dopaminergic neurons of the substantia nigra help regulate motion; they make our physical movements smooth and accurate, so that with practice a ballet dancer can perform beautiful pirouettes and a talented golfer can sink a difficult putt, but also so that one's handwriting can be smooth and legible. Dopaminergic neurons help accomplish that by fine-tuning muscle tone and closely regulating the speed of motion. When too many of these neurons die, a person's everyday motions—such as walking, talking, swallowing, and writing—are affected. Because of the imbalance of muscle tone, tremors may also appear. It is estimated that by the time a person develops the symptoms of Parkinson's, she or he has already lost about 75–80 percent of the dopaminergic neurons in the substantia nigra.

These dopaminergic neurons use dopamine to communicate messages to a part of the brain called the **striatum**. The striatum plays a pivotal role in managing movement. Once a person decides to move an arm or leg, the motor centers of the brain notify the striatum, whose job is to adjust the tone of the various muscles that are involved in the movement. The striatum also determines the force with which these muscles need to contract and the speed and order with which the muscles will have to be activated so that the movement is executed smoothly and with precision. For the striatum to achieve all this, it collects information from all over the body—including the muscles, joints, eyes, and ears—about the locations of arms, legs, hands, feet and their relation to the space and objects surrounding us. Even simple tasks require the brain to make an amazing number of calculations and communication between the brain and the body to be nearly instantaneous. Washing a bowl in a sink of bubbly water requires the brain and body, working together, to calculate water temperature; to pick up a sponge, scrub, and rinse; to examine the cleanliness of the bowl; to put the bowl on a drying rack; and to take care of many other details of the task that we don't even think about.

While all of this is taking place, the substantia nigra neurons use dopamine to help "fine-tune" the neurons that live in the striatum by adjusting their level of excitability (receptiveness to new information). The nerve fibers of the dopamine neurons in the substantia nigra accomplish this function by delivering small amounts of dopamine through their connections, called synapses, to the neurons of the striatum. Dopamine exerts a "push" action on some nerve cells, and a "pull" action on others, and ths "push/pull" action helps "fine tune" the striatum neurons. This fine-tuning is lost when the dopamine neurons of the substantia nigra degenerate, as is the case in Parkinson disease. A person's movements then become less smooth, stiffer (rigidity), and slower (bradykinesia), and the movements appear more hesitant and deliberate, as if "the brakes are on," throughout any type of voluntary movement.

What Causes Parkinson Disease?

Lewy Bodies

We do not know exactly what kills substantia nigra neurons. However, if we look at the substantia nigra of a Parkinson's patient under a microscope we see an accumulation of material inside the bodies of those neurons that have been affected by the disease process. This accumulated material is called Lewy bodies and consists of clogged clumps of damaged proteins (see Figure 2–2). One of the main damaged proteins that accumulates in Lewy bodies is called **synuclein**. This fact is important, because some of the genetic forms of Parkinson disease involve an abnormal gene that results

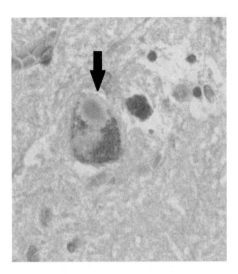

FIGURE 2-2 Interior of a dopaminergic neuron from the substantia nigra of a Parkinson's patient. The round object by the arrow is a Lewy body.

in production of an abnormal form of synuclein. The abnormally formed synuclein molecules have a greater tendency to aggregate and form Lewy bodies.

Lewy bodies are accumulations of abnormal and aged proteins found inside dopaminergic neurons of Parkinson patients.

Another protein seen in the Lewy bodies is called **ubiquitin**. This fact is also important, because in some other hereditary forms of Parkinson's, an abnormal gene causes ubiquitin to function abnormally. Ubiquitin's role has to do with the breakup and elimination of damaged and aged proteins inside neurons. One of the theories as to why substantia nigra neurons die in Parkinson disease hypothesizes that the inability to process old and damaged proteins leads to their accumulation inside the neuron and its eventual demise due to their toxic effects.

Ask the Experts: What Is a Lewy Body?

Dr. Martha Nance says: "The Lewy body is something that the pathologist can see inside the degenerating nerve cells in the brain of a person with Parkinson disease or the related condition **Lewy body disease***. Dr. Frederick Lewy was the neurologist who first identified abnormal blobs of protein inside the degenerating cells in the brains of people with Parkinson disease. People who have Lewy body disease, a more complicated condition that includes not only a Parkinson-like movement disorder but also cognitive changes (dementia) and hallucinations, have many more Lewy bodies than people who just have Parkinson disease.*

"Scientists are currently trying to determine whether Lewy bodies cause damage to the nerve cell or whether they reflect the cell's best efforts to clean up the mess. There is increasing evidence that the Lewy body contains 'worn-out' proteins that should be handled by the cell's recycling system (called the **proteasome***). It seems that one of the things that happen in Parkinson disease is that the proteasome gets overwhelmed and can't keep up, and protein 'trash' collects inside the cell. The Lewy body may represent the cell's attempt to 'sweep the trash into the corner' so that the cell can keep functioning.*

"Two of the genes that have been implicated in Parkinson disease are important in the recycling pathway. **Parkin** *is a protein that is responsible for 'tagging' proteins to be moved to the proteasome for recycling. A mutation in the gene for parkin, then,*

(Continued)

(*Continued*)

interferes with the recycling process and allows the protein trash to accumulate in the cells. Synuclein is one of the main proteins found in the Lewy body. Mutations in the gene for synuclein can cause hereditary Parkinson disease; one could imagine that a mutation in the synuclein gene would lead to the production of a faulty synuclein protein, which would in turn end up in the trash pile sooner than a normal synuclein protein.

"In addition, at least in the test tube, exposure to herbicides and to heavy metals such as manganese and aluminum increases the tendency of synuclein to form protein clumps. Perhaps— nobody knows this for sure—this has something to do with the increased risk of Parkinson disease in welders and farmers.

"Why some people develop Lewy bodies in a small area of the brain (Parkinson disease) while others seem to have a much broader distribution of Lewy bodies even early in their disease course (Lewy body disease) is entirely unknown."

Other Theories About the Cause of Parkinson Disease

There are many more theories about what causes Parkinson disease, and in the following paragraphs we discuss some prominent examples. One theory centers on oxidative stress. Like other cells in our body, neurons use oxygen to produce energy to survive and function properly. The chemical reactions that happen inside cells to extract energy from oxygen molecules produce by-products called **free radicals**, which can damage nerve cells. Neurons normally have the ability to neutralize free radicals and so protect themselves from damage. **Antioxidants** (such as vitamins C and E) are chemicals that boost this neutralizing ability of cells. (Since this effect of antioxidants is not limited to neurons, they are always under consideration when the subject of a cure for Parkinson disease comes up.) In fact, oxidation—the chemical process through which energy is produced from oxygen—is considered an important cause of aging. That is why antioxidants are very popular not only as nutritional supplements for persons with neurodegenerative diseases but also as components of products touted as "anti-aging" remedies. In the context of Parkinson disease, the theory of oxidative stress postulates that there is a breakdown in the ability of the dopaminergic neurons to process an excess amount of toxic free radicals, which in turn leads to their death.

Another popular theory centers on mitochondrial dysfunction. **Mitochondria** are small particles inside the neurons that capture energy from oxygen molecules so that it can be used for the cell's metabolic processes (the constant renewal of the cell's components). These processes are necessary for the ongoing function and survival of the neuron. Many studies have shown that there is some degree of mitochondrial dysfunction in neurons and other cells of persons with Parkinson disease. So it's possible that the demise of the substantia nigra neurons results from the reduced ability of mitochondria to use oxygen efficiently. This has led to further speculation that some nutritional supplements that may improve mitochondrial function may also help slow the progression of Parkinson's. One such supplement, coenzyme Q10, had shown promise for slowing the disease's progression in a few early small studies. However, a very large study, funded by the National Institutes of Health, could not confirm the usefulness of this supplement in slowing down Parkinson's progression.

Processing of iron in the striatum and the substantia nigra can also produce excessive free radicals inside the dopaminergic neurons and thereby contribute to their early demise. Modern research techniques involving the use of **magnetic resonance imaging (MRI)** machines with very powerful magnets have provided measurements indicating that at least in some forms of Parkinson's, there is increased iron content in the striatum and the substantia nigra. Such measurements have supported a role for iron in the genesis of Parkinson disease, but a lot more research is needed before we fully understand the importance of such a connection.

Inflammation in the brain has also been considered as a cause for the loss of dopaminergic neurons. Some infectious diseases, including lethargic encephalitis, West Nile encephalitis, and mycoplasma pneumonia, can cause inflammation in the brain that may damage neurons, including those in the substantia nigra. Physicians have a long tradition of trying anti-inflammatory medications as treatments for neurodegenerative diseases. A group of scientists from the University of Washington recently published a critical review of 11 studies on the relationship between the use of anti-inflammatories and the risk for developing Parkinson disease. They concluded that these studies collectively supported the notion that regular use of these drugs was associated with a slightly lower probability of developing Parkinson disease. A word of caution: Such "observational" studies are usually able to demonstrate associations; however, they cannot establish a cause-and-effect relationship. This means that it does not necessarily follow from these studies that taking anti-inflammatories is a good thing for people with Parkinson's or people who are at risk of getting the disease. Such studies do, however, lend support to the idea that inflammation may be one of the mechanisms that cause Parkinson disease.

This list of possible explanations of neuronal damage in Parkinson disease is by no means inclusive. New theories are published frequently in medical journals and usually have considerable scientific merit. To test such theories, scientists have developed several animal models of Parkinson disease—that is, procedures that produce symptoms like those of Parkinson's in nonhuman animals. Unfortunately, none of the models fully replicates how Parkinson's develops in people. Any conclusions drawn from such laboratory studies continue to be hypothetical and need to be examined further to see whether they apply to people as well as to rats or monkeys.

> Doctors use the **Hoehn and Yahr scale** to report the degree of disease progression and the **Unified Parkinson's Disease Rating Scale** to describe the severity of the symptoms and signs of Parkinson disease.

What Are the Stages of the Disease?

All the theories discussed so far are centered on the substantia nigra, which is in the brainstem. New research shows that the disease process affects other parts of the brain even before it reaches the substantia nigra. This discovery has led scientists to examine the progress of the disease by conducting autopsies to track the pathologic "staging" of Parkinson disease. By looking at the autopsied brains of Parkinson's patients, scientists can judge from the distribution of the Lewy bodies the extent of the disease. Professor Heiko Braak of the Johann Wolfgang Goethe University in Frankfurt, Germany, developed a way of staging the disease based on the extent of pathologic changes in the brains of deceased Parkinson's patients.

However, when determining the disease stage on the basis of clinical symptoms and findings, doctors do not have the benefit of examining the patient's brain under the microscope. In 1967, Drs. Margaret Hoehn and Melvin Yahr developed a staging system for Parkinson disease based on motor symptoms. This five-stage measurement tool gives physicians and patients a rough idea of the progress of the disease. Here's a brief description of the Hoehn and Yahr stages of Parkinson disease:

- **Stage 1:** Persons with Parkinson disease have symptoms only on one side of the body, such as a tremor or some rigidity and slowness of movement in one arm or leg (or both, if on the same side of the body).

- **Stage 2:** Symptoms appear on both sides of the body or in the midline of the body, such as decreased facial expression, drooling, stooping, or shuffling while walking. However, there are no problems with balance. The first two stages are considered "early" or mild.
- **Stage 3:** As soon as a person begins having trouble with balance, she or he has crossed into Stage 3. In this stage, patients don't need help walking or getting up from a sitting position, but their body movements are becoming increasingly slow. The disease is now considered to be mild to moderate.
- **Stage 4:** A person with Parkinson's can no longer be completely independent. Symptoms, including disabling slowness of movement and stiffness, are moderate to severe. The disease's impact on balance and walking is so great that the person usually needs help—from another person or an assistive device—to walk. However, the person is still able to get up from bed or from a chair without help.
- **Stage 5:** Once a person with Parkinson's is unable to get up from a bed or chair without help, they have crossed into Stage 5. The person requires help or even nursing care for the majority of daily activities.

Thanks to **levodopa**—our most effective drug to treat the symptoms of Parkinson disease—determining how far the disease has progressed has become more complex. As an example, when a patient is taking medications he or she may qualify for a Stage 2 rating, but when the medications don't work the same person may function only at the level of Stage 4.

Neurologists also use a standardized scoring system in order to rate the severity (as opposed to the stage) of the motor symptoms of Parkinson disease. Titled the Unified Parkinson's Disease Rating Scale (UPDRS), this system was developed in the 1980s and has been revised most recently by the Movement Disorder Society, an international association of neurologists specializing in the treatment of Parkinson disease and other movement disorders. The UPDRS consists of a number of questions and an examination. The answers to the questions as well as the severity of the signs of the disease found during the examination are rated, for the most part on a scale of 0 to 4. The sum of these ratings is the UPDRS score. This is a useful way to measure a patient's progress from visit to visit and to assess when medications work or don't work. However, the scale has limitations for comparing the severity of the illness of different patients. The same score in two patients may actually be associated with different degrees of severity and different types of symptoms and impairment.

> **Age**, **genetics**, and **environmental exposures** may all contribute to a person's risk of coming down with Parkinson disease.

Who Gets the Disease? Why Me?

When diagnosed with an illness, one of the first questions people ask is straightforward: "Why me?" For Parkinson disease, as with most diseases affecting the brain, the answer is not simple. Age, genetics, and exposure to certain environmental conditions may be risk factors in the development of Parkinson disease, but no single thing is known to be its cause. In the next few paragraphs we'll explore risk factors that may contribute to a person's developing Parkinson disease.

Age is one of the leading factors associated with the risk of coming down with Parkinson's. Older people are more likely to have the disease than the young. Close to 1.5 million people are currently living with Parkinson disease in the United States, and approximately

50,000 Americans are diagnosed with the disease every year; most of them are over the age of 60. However, people as young as 20 or older than 100 may develop Parkinson's. The aging of the "baby boomer" generation is expected to boost the number of people living with Parkinson disease, which is the second most common neurodegenerative disease after Alzheimer disease. Statistics suggest that Parkinson disease strikes men slightly more often than women (approximately six men get Parkinson's for every four women who are diagnosed with the disease) and that it is slightly more frequent among Caucasians than among Africans, Asians, and Native Americans.

Another risk factor is genetics. Scientific research indicates that anywhere between 5 and 15 percent of Parkinson's patients inherited the disease itself or the tendency to develop it. With the development of the science of genetics in recent decades, variants of a number of genes have been identified that cause Parkinson disease; this has contributed greatly to our understanding of the mechanisms of the disease. For most of our genes, we inherit two copies, one from our father and one from our mother. Some of these inherited genes are *dominant*, which means that we need only one "abnormal" copy to get the disease. With dominant genes, then, one of the parents has to have the abnormal gene—and therefore the disease—for a child to get it too. Other genes are *recessive*. Recessive genes require a person to have two abnormal copies to get the disease: one from the father and one from the mother. In this case, the person's parents both carry the abnormal gene but neither one may actually have Parkinson disease, since each may have only one copy of the abnormal gene. Some of the most discussed genes associated with the hereditary forms of Parkinson disease are the alpha-synuclein gene (also called SNCA), the dardarin gene (or LRRK-2), the parkin gene (PARK2), and the glucocerebrosidase gene. Patients who contract Parkinson's at a younger age are more likely to have a genetic abnormality at the root of their disease.

Ask the Experts: Is Parkinson Disease Hereditary?

Dr. Demetrius Maraganore says: "In the classical sense, Parkinson disease is not hereditary. Since the mid-1800s, doctors have observed that people with Parkinson disease often have relatives who also develop Parkinson disease. In fact, 15–20 percent of people living with Parkinson disease also have relatives with the ailment. But that doesn't mean the illness is hereditary. More than one family member can have a sore throat or tuberculosis, but that doesn't mean that sore throats or tuberculosis is hereditary.

"To determine the prevalence of Parkinson disease in families, researchers have conducted several large studies involving hundreds of people with Parkinson disease and hundreds of people without the disease. The studies found that if you don't have a relative with Parkinson disease, your lifetime risk for the disease is about 2 percent. If you have a relative with Parkinson disease, your lifetime risk for the disease is about 4 percent. That's still a very low risk.

"In recent years, scientists have studied the human genome. When it comes to Parkinson disease, there are only a few gene variations that contribute to an increased risk for acquiring the disease. For people with those gene variations, the lifetime risk of contracting the disease increases from 2 percent to 2.4 percent. The gene that is most convincingly associated with increased risk for Parkinson disease in populations worldwide is the alpha-synuclein (SNCA) gene. Other susceptibility genes include MAPT and LRRK-2, but their contributions to Parkinson disease affect some populations more than others.

"There are also gene mutations that can outright cause Parkinson disease, albeit rarely. The affected genes include SNCA,

(Continued)

> (*Continued*)
> *Parkin, UCHL1, DJ1, PINK1, and LRRK-2. Specific mutations in these genes can cause multiple people in the same family to get Parkinson disease.* "After decades of research, the scientific conclusion is that the bulk of what causes Parkinson disease does not appear to be genetic, and we are largely in the dark about specific causes of the disease."

Another risk factor is exposure to certain environmental conditions. Studies have shown that people with long-term exposure to some organic solvents, pesticides, and herbicides are at higher risk of developing Parkinson disease. People who live in rural areas and drink well water most of their lives or who live near wood-pulp-processing plants are also at higher risk of contracting Parkinson's. However, most people with Parkinson disease never had exposure to these environmental conditions, and most people who were exposed don't get Parkinson's.

> Exposure to **paraquat**, a pesticide, triples the risk of getting Parkinson disease.

Some occupations also have been associated with a higher risk of Parkinson disease, including farming, teaching, anesthesiology, and welding (although there are some conflicting studies on this latter one). There are several theories about why these people in these occupations are vulnerable to Parkinson disease. For example, manganese poisoning, which can cause symptoms similar to Parkinson's, has been offered as a possible explanation for welders' raised risk, and pesticide exposure for that of farmers. However, there is no definitive explanation for any of these occupational associations.

Ask the Experts: Do Chemicals Cause Parkinson Disease?

Dr. *Demetrius Maraganore says: "Doctors and some patients have wondered whether exposure to certain chemicals causes Parkinson disease or a Parkinson-like illness. The research on this question hasn't resulted in a direct correlation between any specific chemical and Parkinson's or a Parkinson-like illness. It's very difficult to prove that short- or long-term exposure to a chemical caused Parkinson disease decades later.*

"However, sometimes a chemical appears to cause Parkinson-like symptoms very quickly. **MPTP** *is a neurotoxin. In the 1980s, a group of drug addicts injected MPTP-laced heroin into their bodies and quickly developed* **parkinsonism**— *symptoms similar to those of Parkinson disease. In 1996, William Langston wrote about this in his book* The Case of the Frozen Addicts. *This case led scientists to wonder if MPTP might be the cause of Parkinson's. So researchers injected monkeys with MPTP, who also rapidly developed Parkinson-like symptoms.*

"MPTP has a similar chemical makeup to paraquat, a poisonous herbicide used to kill grass and weeds. Since MPTP causes parkinsonism, researchers wondered whether paraquat also might cause Parkinson disease. This triggered two decades of scientific research focusing on whether farmers, gardeners, and other people exposed to paraquat or other pesticides had higher rates of Parkinson disease than the population as a whole. The results: Most people with Parkinson's didn't have exposure to pesticides, and most people with exposure to pesticides don't develop Parkinson disease. At best, pesticides may be a contributing factor to contracting the disease, but the effect is small.

(Continued)

(Continued)

"Another chemical that has been studied is manganese, which is found in welding rods. When welders melt welding rods, a gas containing manganese is released. Breathing too much of this manganese-containing gas may be harmful. There have been instances of welders experiencing the symptoms associated with Parkinson disease at an early age. When this happens it is called manganism. This possible link to Parkinson's demands further study. These observations also emphasize the importance of welders' using protective equipment to prevent exposures to harmful fumes."

Researchers have also studied whether certain infections or severe head injuries can make a person more likely to contract Parkinson disease. No particular infection has been consistently associated with Parkinson's, although a number of brain infections can cause illnesses that resemble Parkinson disease: the most notable infection causing signs similar to Parkinson disease is lethargic encephalitis, also known as the sleeping sickness. Likewise, studies examining a possible connection between head injuries and Parkinson disease have proved inconclusive. In a recently presented study, Dr. Samuel Goldman reported that some people who have one particular variant of the alpha-synuclein gene (a gene some of whose abnormal variants can cause a hereditary form of Parkinson), have a higher risk for developing Parkinson's after head injuries than people who do not possess that variant.

The "**loaded gun**" **theory** of the cause of Parkinson disease postulates that a person's genetic makeup "loads the gun" but that some environmental factor is necessary to "pull the trigger."

Ask the Experts: Do Smoking and Caffeine Protect Against Parkinson Disease?

Dr. Demetrius Maraganore says: "For decades, researchers have noticed that people with Parkinson disease are more likely to be nonsmokers than the general public.

"One theory about why smokers seem less likely to contract Parkinson disease centered on the relationship between smoking and dopamine. Smoking stimulates dopamine transmission in the brain, and dopamine transmission creates a sensation of pleasure or reward. Most addictive substances act on dopamine transmission. However, Parkinson disease patients have less dopamine as a result of dopamine neuron degeneration. Hence, smoking may have less effect on the depleted dopamine systems of persons destined to develop Parkinson disease and thus may trigger less pleasure or reward (and hence less likelihood to smoke or to become addicted).

"Clinicians have also noticed that people with Parkinson disease are less likely to drink coffee than the general population. This has raised the question of whether coffee protects against the disease. Alternatively, it may be that reduced coffee use in persons destined to develop Parkinson disease is due to reduced pleasure or reward, as for smoking."

Is There Help?

Nearly four years after Count de Lordat was diagnosed with the disease, James Parkinson described the man this way: "He still walked alone with a cane, from one room to the other, but with great difficulty, and in a tottering manner; his left hand and arm were much reduced, and would hardly perform any motion; the right was somewhat benumbed, and he could scarcely lift up his head; his saliva was continually trickling out of his mouth, and he had neither the power of retaining it, nor of spitting it out freely." Fortunately, modern medicine has considerably improved the lives of Parkinson patients, and the count would have done much better today.

Insights on how to treat Parkinson disease with medications didn't emerge until the mid-20th century, when physicians noticed that schizophrenia patients on antipsychotic drugs began developing symptoms of Parkinson disease. So researchers began examining possible relationships between the antipsychotic drugs and the cause of Parkinson disease. These scientists discovered that the antipsychotic drugs deprived the brain of the effects of dopamine. Pathologists already knew that the substantia nigra appeared very pale in the brains of people who had died of Parkinson disease, in contrast to normal brains, where it had an intense blue-black hue. As it turns out, the neurons of the substantia nigra produce dopamine, and dopamine turns black when it's packaged for storage inside these cells. Putting two and two together, scientists realized that the loss of dopamine in the brainstem was the cause of the symptoms of Parkinson disease.

So why not just give Parkinson's patients dopamine pills to replace the loss of dopamine in the brain? Doctors did that, but there was a problem. Without a healthy brain, the body can't function, so the brain has a kind of protective shield called the **blood–brain barrier**. This barrier is a system of specialized cells and processes designed to keep the brain safe from toxins and infections. The blood–brain barrier is therefore a very good thing, but it does make it trickier for doctors to help patients with brain disorders like Parkinson disease, because dopamine cannot cross it.

In 1968, Dr. George C. Cotzias published a scientific article in the *New England Journal of Medicine* titled "Levodopa for Parkinsonism." Based on laboratory research, Cotzias suggested treating Parkinson's patients with high doses of levodopa (or L-dopa) because levodopa crosses the blood–brain barrier and the neurons can convert levodopa into dopamine. Although doctors had already tried this approach without success, Dr. Cotzias used the drug at much higher dosages than the ones that had been previously tried. Once levodopa crosses the blood–brain barrier and is inside the brain, it reaches the brainstem and gets transformed into dopamine, temporarily enabling Parkinson's patients to regain control and fluidity of their movements while also reducing tremor and muscle stiffness.

Awakenings, a 1990 film starring Robin Williams and Robert De Niro, was based on real patient stories taken from a book in which Dr. Oliver Sacks described the impact of levodopa on patients who had had Parkinson's symptoms for many years.

The introduction of levodopa to treat Parkinson disease in 1968 generated optimism among neurologists that there really was an effective treatment for Parkinson disease. Unfortunately, levodopa doesn't cure Parkinson's; it merely treats its symptoms, causing temporary relief from the long-term, debilitating effects of the illness. As the disease progresses, damage spreads to other neurons that are *not* dependent on dopamine for their function. When this happens, Parkinson's patients may develop symptoms that are not improved by enhancing the dopamine content of the brain. Nonetheless, researchers like Dr. Ryan Uitti of the Mayo Clinic in Jacksonville, Florida, have demonstrated that the introduction of levodopa has dramatically increased the life spans of persons living with Parkinson's. It comes as no surprise that levodopa is considered one of the greatest breakthroughs in medical therapeutics in the 20th century.

In the 1970s and 1980s, research on medication for Parkinson's focused on optimizing the use of levodopa and minimizing the drug's side effects. The resulting advances allowed people to live fuller, longer lives, but they also presented a challenge. As people with Parkinson disease lived longer, the disease began affecting parts of the brain that were spared in earlier stages. Early in its course, Parkinson disease affects how well people can walk, talk, write, and perform other daily activities. Later in the disease, however, it can also affect thinking and cause unexplained falling, confusion, or fainting, which are symptoms that not only do not respond to additional dopamine but may in fact get worse from it.

The Outlook for Parkinson's Patients

The prognosis of Parkinson disease has changed considerably over the years. Before the advent of levodopa and other effective treatments for the motor symptoms of Parkinson disease, the average survival after diagnosis was approximately five years. (This means that about 50 percent of people diagnosed with Parkinson disease died within five years.) The average survival after diagnosis has since improved dramatically. Today, it is calculated that on average the life expectancy of a person with Parkinson disease is approximately one-and-a-half to two years less than that of people without the disease. It is not unusual for many people who have lived with Parkinson disease for years to die "with" rather than "from" Parkinson's. However, survival varies dramatically among patients.

Some people experience a quick and aggressive form of the disease. In other people, the disease makes only slow and subtle changes to the body, so that they do not experience much decline is from one year to the next. About one in 10 Parkinson's patients has a very benign version of the disease and experiences very slow progression. It so happens that patients that have a more benign course tend to have more tremors when first diagnosed with the disease. This has led some experts to distinguish these patients as having **benign tremulous parkinsonism**. Patients with a younger age of onset have a better overall prognosis in terms of survival and the ability to retain the benefits from anti-Parkinson medications. However, younger patients also have a greater chance of experiencing treatment complications.

Our ability to treat the motor symptoms of Parkinson disease is better now than, say, 50 years ago, but extending the life expectancy of people with Parkinson disease has led to some unforeseen consequences. Since people with Parkinson disease now live longer, the disease spreads further in their brains, causing more and more symptoms for which we have not yet found very good treatments. Researchers now believe that about one in three people with Parkinson disease will end up developing dementia. In addition, about one in three people with Parkinson disease will end up having to use a walker, wheelchair, or other gait assistive device. Patients with Parkinson disease are more likely to be admitted to a nursing home than the general population.

Over the past few years, specialists treating Parkinson's patients have become increasingly aware of these problems and have turned their attention to new research designed to address problems and symptoms that emerge in the later stages of the disease and for which no effective treatment is yet available. This line of research is almost as important as the line of research looking for a cure for the disease or for medications that may slow down its progression. If researchers can find treatments that will not only prolong the life of Parkinson's patients but also eliminate problems that diminish their quality of life, then finding a cure may become less critical.

In parallel with research geared toward improving the quality of life of advanced Parkinson's patients, research efforts are increasingly focused on slowing the progression of the disease and finding a cure for it. New hope for a cure has been spurred by our increasingly detailed understanding of the processes that lead to premature neuronal death. This new information has been provided by recent advances in genetics and stem cell research. New approaches to testing new pharmaceuticals as possible curative agents may eliminate the need for very long, elaborate, and expensive drug trials while dramatically increasing the number of drugs that can be tested simultaneously. Cross-pollination with ideas, theories, and experimental data from research on other neurodegenerative diseases (such as Alzheimer disease) or even from basic research in disciplines as diverse as chemical engineering and nanotechnology, greatly facilitated by the widespread use of the Internet, has opened new avenues to explore. There is general optimism among Parkinson disease specialists that drugs that treat the disease itself, not just the symptoms, and even a cure may not be that far off.

Chapter 3

The Motor Symptoms

Dr. James Parkinson first described in 1817 (nearly 200 years ago!) what have become known as the classic symptoms of Parkinson disease: tremor, rigidity (muscle stiffness), and bradykinesia (slowness of movement). To these three symptoms, modern neurologists have added the "loss of postural correcting reflexes" (balance trouble). A great many of the motor difficulties patients notice can be explained as manifestations of these four so-called cardinal symptoms. For example, micrographia, the small and scrawny handwriting that many Parkinson's patients have, is really a manifestation of bradykinesia. In this and the next chapter, we'll explore and explain common and not-so-common symptoms that people living with Parkinson's develop throughout the course of the disease.

A person with Parkinson disease may not have all four cardinal symptoms. For example, one in four people with the disease never experiences tremor. There is only one exception to this rule: bradykinesia. According to the most accepted set of diagnostic criteria for Parkinson disease, bradykinesia has to be present or the diagnosis cannot be made with a reasonable degree of certainty. That is, a person cannot be diagnosed with Parkinson disease unless he or she exhibits bradykinesia. By itself, however, bradykinesia is not sufficient to establish the diagnosis. One of the other three cardinal symptoms also has to be present.

This list of four symptoms does not by any means describe the whole spectrum of motor symptoms of Parkinson disease. Many patients may have other motor symptoms not explained by these four main symptoms, such as **dystonia**, the abnormal simultaneous contraction of muscles normally having opposing functions, or motor symptoms related to their medications, such as **dyskinesias**, which are erratic, involuntary movements of the arm, leg, trunk, or face muscles. The following sections describe and explain the various motor symptoms of the disease, including some of the more unusual ones, and discuss their potential impact on people's lives.

Tremor

Tremor is the most visible symptom of Parkinson's. For many people, whether they have the disease or not, any experience of tremor raises the worry, "Do I have Parkinson's?" The tremor has been such a fixture of the disease in people's imaginations that James Parkinson's name for it, "the shaking palsy," remains very much in use. Yet as mentioned earlier, not everyone with Parkinson disease gets tremors. (About 20–25 percent of Parkinson's patients never experience tremors.)

Tremor usually shows up first in one arm or leg and may even affect only a single finger. It is more likely to happen when the arm or leg is resting, then stop or subside as soon as the person moves the arm or leg. Therefore it's often called rest or resting tremor. The arm or leg may begin shaking at times of increased stress, fear, or anger or in other emotional situations. It may appear only when people are walking with the arm dangling on their side. Sometimes it may give the impression that the person is rubbing something between the thumb and pointer finger. (That's why the name "pill-rolling tremor" is sometimes used.) As time passes and the disease worsens, the tremor may be more persistent, appear even with movement of the arm or leg, spread to bigger muscles of the affected limb, or appear in other limbs as well. It generally remains most severe in the arm or leg where it started.

Tremors have a somewhat unusual relationship with the progression of the disease and often change over time. Thus in some people, tremor may be the main symptom at the beginning of the disease and then dissipate or even disappear as the disease worsens. In others tremor may be very severe from the start and not respond well to medications. Interestingly, the presence of tremor early on is a good prognostic sign, which is to say that people with a "tremor-predominant" clinical picture tend to do better over the years than patients who have no tremor at the time of diagnosis. Drs. Margaret Hoehn and Melvin Yahr reported their study on the natural progression of Parkinson disease in 1967, just before levodopa was used as a very effective treatment of the symptoms. After reviewing the cases of 802 patients, they concluded that "at least during the first ten years of the illness, parkinsonism with tremor as the initial symptom progresses more slowly than parkinsonism with other heralding symptoms." Neurologists sometimes use the term "benign tremulous parkinsonism" to describe patients who have mostly a rest tremor with few, if any, other symptoms of the disease.

> **Tremor** at the time of diagnosis may be a sign of a more benign course. However, it is not always fully controlled with drugs.

Tremor can be difficult to treat and may be disabling. Although most Parkinson disease medications are quite effective in controlling or even fully eliminating tremor, they don't always work. Approximately one in five Parkinson patients may have "treatment-resistant" tremor, which means that the tremor cannot be fully or even partially controlled with medications.

Bradykinesia

Bradykinesia is a Greek word that means "slow movement." According to the most widely accepted diagnostic criteria for Parkinson's, if bradykinesia is not present, a diagnosis of Parkinson disease cannot be made with certainty. Although the term implies slowness, it also refers to the size of the movements. Not only do people living with Parkinson disease move slower, but their movements are also smaller. So when a neurologist examines how fast a patient can tap the pointer finger and the thumb against each other, the doctor is looking at how big those movements are as well as the speed of the movement. Many patients will make progressively smaller movements when asked to perform the task repeatedly.

> In the absence of **bradykinesia** (slow movements) a doctor cannot make the diagnosis of Parkinson disease.

This slowing and size reduction in movements may show itself in several ways. Handwriting often becomes smaller, and it takes more time to write words. Many people also experience a loss of arm swing when walking. Other examples of bradykinesia include loss of facial expression with less blinking of the eyes (the "mask face"), slurred speech, soft voice, loss of manual dexterity, difficulty getting up from a low chair, and shuffling of steps while walking.

Bradykinesia also affects reaction time. A Parkinson's patient who trips while walking may fall because he or she isn't quick enough to recover balance. Bradykinesia may have been the cause of the tripping in the first place: persons with Parkinson's don't lift their feet high enough to clear obstacles when walking. Bradykinesia is also the reason that people with Parkinson disease may have difficulty getting up from a low seat, getting in and out of a car, and getting in and out of bed. In the early stages, bradykinesia usually happens on either the right or left side of a person. But over time it will spread to the other side as well.

Medications used to treat the motor symptoms of Parkinson disease are quite effective with bradykinesia, especially in the early stages of the illness. Additionally, special exercises have been developed to address this particular problem. These treatments are discussed in detail in Chapters 7, 8, and 9.

Rigidity

Rigidity is the medical term for stiffness. Our muscles are never fully relaxed, but they maintain a level of muscle tone when at rest. This "rest" muscle tone is increased in patients with Parkinson disease. Just like tremor and bradykinesia, this symptom is worse on one side of the body than the other. People may experience rigidity as muscle tightness, but they may also experience it as a painful, cramplike sensation in the muscles or as muscle spasms. Sometimes an achy, tired feeling may be the only indication of rigidity, and often, in the earliest stages, Parkinson's patients may be misdiagnosed as having a pinched nerve in their neck or their lower back. In more advanced stages, rigidity may cause an uncomfortable feeling in the muscles of the chest or of the abdominal wall, which sometimes leads to emergency consultations to rule out a heart attack. Some Parkinson's patients with these symptoms go through many tests and consultations with gastroenterologists to look for ulcers or other intestinal conditions. A word of caution is necessary here: Although many unusual sensations and symptoms can be attributed to Parkinson disease, Parkinson's patients are vulnerable to cardiac (heart) and gastrointestinal (digestive system) conditions just like everyone else. So they should not just blame any new and unusual symptoms on Parkinson disease without discussing them with their doctor first.

> **Rigidity** is an increase in muscle tone that makes people with Parkinson disease look stiff.

Rigidity also contributes to a decrease in the size of hand, arm, and leg movements by decreasing flexibility. This is why many people living with the disease appear stiff when walking, turning, or getting up from a lying or sitting position. Because rigidity causes the muscles to be shorter when at rest, it may also lead to a "flexed" attitude of the arms, legs, or entire body. This effect results in a stooped posture or a sideways lean when standing. This stooping and leaning is called **camptocormia**, which is Greek for "crooked trunk."

Rigidity responds favorably, particularly early on, to drugs. However, sometimes patients may continue to have muscle spasms because of rigidity even when all other symptoms are under control. For this reason special exercises, including stretching and dancing, are often recommended for Parkinson patients. Details on this type of treatment are to be found in Chapter 8.

Loss of Balance, Freezing, and Falling

People living with Parkinson disease may experience a loss of balance for a variety of reasons, but this problem usually happens in the moderate to advanced stages of the disease. The classic teaching is that balance is not an issue for people recently diagnosed with Parkinson disease. But this statement needs to be taken with a grain of salt. It is well known that 20–25 percent of all people over the age of 65 will experience repeated falls. Thus losing one's balance is not unusual in the age group that is most likely to be living with Parkinson disease.

Here is a more accurate statement: In the early stages of the disease, patients are not likely to lose their balance because of Parkinson disease. However, they may be more likely to trip, not be quick enough to catch themselves, and therefore fall. It is important to point out that *frequent* falls early in the course of the disease should be brought to the doctor's attention, because they may indicate that Parkinson disease is not the correct diagnosis. More details on this can be found in Chapter 5.

As the disease progresses, three things may happen that will increase the likelihood of falling: loss of postural correcting reflexes, freezing of gait, and orthostatic hypotension.

> There are many reasons why people with Parkinson's may **lose their balance** and fall. Therefore it's always important to discuss falling with the doctor.

Loss of postural correcting reflexes isn't well understood. It is not directly connected to the slowness of reaction that many patients experience, because it sometimes happens to people whose bradykinesia is under excellent control with medication. When this symptom occurs, Parkinson's patients tend to lose their balance for no apparent reason. The person may be doing normal things, such as backing up while opening the refrigerator door, or may be in the process of sitting down. Falling backward (a symptom called retropulsion) is a common occurrence in such cases. Doctors will often do a "pull test" to examine the patient's postural correcting reflexes. With the patient standing in front of the doctor, she or he will give a quick, sharp backward tug on the patient's shoulders. If the patient needs to be caught by the doctor to keep from falling, the test is positive. As the disease progresses, falls due to loss of postural correcting reflexes may become so frequent that some people may fall tens of times every day.

An unfortunate characteristic of this symptom is that it rarely disappears with adjustments of anti-Parkinson drugs or with brain surgery. The doctor may ask for help from a physical therapist who can assess the need and appropriateness of a gait assistive device or may refer the patient to an occupational therapist to educate the patient and caregiver on things as simple as how to safely put on one's pants or as complicated as what kind of adaptive equipment should be obtained (rails in hallways, grab bars in bathrooms, etc.). Details on these treatments are contained in Chapter 8.

Freezing of gait describes what happens when a person's feet "get stuck to the ground" while she or he is walking. This symptom appears in the moderate to advanced stages of the disease, and researchers aren't sure what causes it. Freezing of gait may happen as a person first gets up to start walking, but it may also happen in midstride, especially when the person is turning or going through doorways or narrow passages (as at the checkout lane of a grocery store). Interestingly, freezing is less likely to happen on stairs or when there is a striped pattern on the floor. Some walking surfaces, such as uneven ground or carpets, may make the condition more likely to occur. If freezing happens when a person is trying to pivot or jumping up to answer the phone, it can lead to a fall. Although freezing of gait may not respond to anti-Parkinson medications, it may be overcome with certain tricks. A physical therapist can teach patients such techniques, which are described in more detail in Chapters 8 and 9.

People living with Parkinson disease sometimes fall as a result of **orthostatic hypotension** (also called postural hypotension). This medical term means that on arising, a person's blood pressure drops precipitously (see Chapter 4 for greater detail). Parkinson disease affects the autonomic nervous system, which is the part of the nervous system that controls functions of our body that are not under voluntary control, such as stomach and intestinal motility, beating of the heart, and production of sweat and saliva. The autonomic nervous system is also in charge of making sure our blood pressure remains stable when we stand up from a reclining or sitting position. We all have experienced a woozy sensation if we get up too fast, especially if we are a little dehydrated or have been kneeling or bending over. This happens because when we stand up, our blood, responding to gravity, has a tendency to pool in our legs; this can cause less blood to travel to the brain. When this happens, the brain shuts down and we faint. It is the job of the autonomic nervous system to make sure this does not happen by adjusting the tone of the veins in our legs and the force and rate with which our heart pumps blood.

Parkinson disease often affects how well the autonomic nervous system does its job. In addition, many of the anti-Parkinson drugs override the autonomic nervous system's responses, creating a perfect storm that can result in fainting or near fainting. In the advanced stages of the disease, this can result in more falls. In Chapter 7 we discuss medications for orthostatic hypotension, and in Chapter 9 we discuss many strategies to minimize the risk of falls and injuries regardless of the cause of falling (which can vary from patient to patient).

Other Motor Symptoms

Weakness

Muscle weakness is not considered a symptom of Parkinson disease. This may be because when doctors test muscle strength manually in a Parkinson's patient, they cannot generally detect such weakness. But some patients report experiencing weakness. They may be perceiving bradykinesia and rigidity as weakness: the person may not be able to generate muscle power quickly enough when performing certain tasks. But it is possible that in some patients there is an actual decrease in strength: some studies conducted with specialized equipment have demonstrated slight reductions in the muscle strength of people living with Parkinson disease. In the more advanced stages of the disease, strength can be decreased further because of decreased use of certain muscles. If left unchecked, such weakness can combine with rigidity to cause muscle atrophy (muscle wasting) and eventually contractures (the development of scar tissue inside the muscles). The result can be fixed positions of the extremities and total loss of elasticity and muscle function. For this reason, even in the most advanced stages of the disease, continued exercise remains an important part of treatment. Health care professionals such as physical and occupational therapists can assess the patients' abilities and needs and advise on the type and extent of the exercises that are likely to be helpful.

Dystonia

Dystonia happens when muscles contract involuntarily. When dystonia occurs, muscles that are supposed to work opposite each other get activated simultaneously—a phenomenon called co-contraction. This leads to cramplike postures and slow, "tense" involuntary movements of the arms, the legs, the trunk, or the face and neck.

Dystonia is a disease in its own right, separate from Parkinson disease. When dystonia happens as a symptom of Parkinson disease, it is called secondary or symptomatic dystonia. Parkinson-related dystonia and dystonic postures may be a symptom of the disease, particularly in younger patients, but may also be experienced as a form of motor fluctuation, similar to dyskinesia (these terms are explained in detail later in this chapter). In the former case, dystonia may happen very early in the morning, when people first wake up and before they take their morning medication, or it may happen when the effect of the drugs "wears off." It may also occur as a side effect of anti-Parkinson medicine, particularly levodopa. When dystonia happens as a motor fluctuation, it may be difficult for the doctor to decide whether more or less medicine is the correct solution. The doctor will ask for a detailed description, and sometimes the patient will be asked to keep detailed diaries of the timing of this symptom, especially in relation to the timing of the medication. The patient may have to come into the clinic and be observed throughout a cycle of the medication over a few hours.

Dystonia can be painful. Early in the disease it usually responds favorably to anti-Parkinson drugs, but later it may not. Sometimes when it appears as a motor fluctuation, it may worsen with medication. In such cases, other medications may need to be added to the treatment, including medications used to treat dystonia the disease. Sometimes, injections of botulinum toxin may be helpful. Dystonia-related pain usually responds to the treatment of the dystonia, but over-the-counter painkillers may also be helpful.

Akinesia

Although akinesia is sometimes singled out as a separate symptom, it often is just bradykinesia "gone wild." The word "akinesia" is Greek for "absence of movement." It is used to describe patients who become suddenly unable to move. Patients with akinesia usually experience it in the moderate to advanced stages of the disease, and it usually happens in the middle of the night, when a person wakes up and is unable to get out of bed without help. That's one of the reasons why doctors may prescribe anti-Parkinson drug doses to be given at bedtime or sometimes in the middle of the night.

Difficulties with Speech, Voice, and Swallowing

Although most people take speech, voice, and swallowing for granted, they are delicately choreographed motor activities that require fine coordination of many muscles. For most of us, these activities have become automatic from many years of practice. One can almost imagine a computer program somewhere in the brain that gets started and runs speech, voice, and swallowing "on autopilot." However, when the neural hardware that's responsible for tuning all these muscles to the proper pitch or muscle tone ceases to work properly or respond fast enough, these otherwise automatic tasks become a struggle.

That's what happens to many people with Parkinson disease. Words become slurred and run together (a problem called **dysarthria**); speech sometimes accelerates and loses its expressiveness. Breathing movements are smaller and the person does not expel enough air to produce a sufficiently loud voice (**dysphonia**). Meaning is not conveyed properly, and as the voice becomes softer and less resonant, it may lose its emotional inflection and content. All these changes, together with loss of facial expression, often make communication very difficult for the Parkinson's patient. Problems communicating become a frequent point of friction in couples as each person blames the other's voice or hearing. A person with Parkinson disease can very effectively correct the problem, especially in the earlier stages, by making a conscious effort to speak loudly and clearly and to separate words. In a way it's like switching from "auto" to "manual." A speech pathologist may be instrumental in teaching patients useful exercises to encourage this practice; details are discussed in Chapters 8 and 9.

Swallowing is affected in a similar fashion (called **dysphagia**). Most people automatically clear their throat at all times by constantly swallowing saliva as well as all secretions that may be running down the back of the throat from the sinuses and the nose cavities. This automatic activity slows down considerably in people with Parkinson disease. As a result, patients may drool and report having thick secretions and feeling like they have a "frog in the throat." Another reason for this annoying sensation is that the many drugs a Parkinson patient may be taking can cause thickening of the saliva. In more advanced stages, the choreography of the swallowing movements may be completely lost and food may not be easily or properly propelled through the esophagus. As a result choking can occur when food and liquid slide down "the wrong pipe" and end up in the trachea (commonly called the windpipe). Besides the obvious danger of choking, in the later stages of the disease dysphagia may lead to aspiration pneumonia (lung infection). When anything other than air goes down the windpipe, one normally starts coughing, forcefully expelling the swallowed item. In the advanced stages of Parkinson disease, this protective cough reflex may be dampened or completely lost, so that foods and liquids may end up in the lungs without the patient's realizing what happened. Such materials may become a breeding ground for bacteria in the lung, which may result in aspiration pneumonia. There are many treatment strategies to deal with swallowing trouble, as discussed in greater detail in Chapters 8 and 9.

Double Vision

Persons with Parkinson disease have many difficulties with their vision, but one frequent symptom is double vision, or **diplopia**. Double vision may happen as a manifestation of various neurologic conditions but can also be part of the natural aging process. When such a problem appears it should be discussed with and assessed by a physician, because it may not be the result of Parkinson's but may indicate another serious condition. In Parkinson disease, double vision arises from the inability of the eyes to keep pace with each other. Normally, each eye sends the brain a slightly different image, because the eyes look at an object from different angles. The brain is capable of fusing the two images into a single, three-dimensional image. When the alignment of the eyes is slightly off, the two images don't merge or they fuse incompletely. In milder cases, this is experienced as a "ghosting" similar to what TV images look like when reception is slightly off. In more severe cases, people see two separate images.

In Parkinson disease, the muscles that move the eyes are do not respond very quickly, and because one side of the body is more affected than the other, the eyes do not move in sync. This may cause double or blurred vision. In addition, some drugs may impair convergence, which is the ability to bring the eyes close together to focus on an object close to the nose. This "convergence insufficiency" can happen normally as we get older, but some anti-Parkinson medications may aggravate it. Other anti-Parkinson medications may reduce the ability of the eye to adjust its focus when looking at objects from afar or close-up. Persons with Parkinson disease tend to not blink as often as is necessary to lubricate the eyes, and this can lead to a thin film of haze over the eyes, which causes blurring of vision. The use of bifocals, trifocals, or progressive lenses may further compound all these problems. Medications are generally not very effective to correct vision trouble, but over-the-counter lubricating eyedrops may be helpful with dryness and associated discomfort. A visit to the eye doctor is necessary if simple measures fail.

Other vision problems besides double vision can pester a person with Parkinson disease. Those will be discussed in the sensory symptoms section in Chapter 4.

Apraxia

Apraxia is an inability of the brain to plan and execute certain movements. The term means "inability to act." Medicine recognizes several types of apraxia, and entire books have been dedicated to this phenomenon. Apraxia is not exclusive to Parkinson disease. It is often seen in people with strokes, traumatic brain injury, and Alzheimer disease and many other degenerative brain diseases. The person affected may give the impression of having forgotten how to perform certain motor tasks. Some specialists believe that freezing of gait, which affects people in the more advanced stages of Parkinson, is a form of apraxia. In apraxia, the failure happens at the highest level of command in a person's brain, the part that plans and initiates specific motor tasks. Since this part of the brain is not affected in Parkinson disease until its later stages, this symptom is usually seen in advanced cases. In fact, appearance of apraxia early on may be an indication that the diagnosis of Parkinson disease is not accurate. Although the most common form of apraxia seen in Parkinson's is freezing of gait, other forms may occasionally be encountered, such as apraxia of eye opening, inability to seat oneself, and inability to use utensils.

Unfortunately, apraxia is very difficult to treat. Sometimes physical and occupational therapy may help the patient to develop alternative techniques. Apraxia has become an area of more intense and focused research in recent years, and there is good reason to believe that more effective rehabilitation techniques will be available soon.

Motor Symptoms That May Occur as a Complication of Treatment

Dyskinesia

"Dyskinesia" is another word derived from Greek. "Dys" means difficult or abnormal, and "kinesis" translates as "movement." Dyskinesia is a word used to describe random-looking involuntary movements. Strictly speaking, dyskinesia is not a symptom of Parkinson disease. The term is used to describe the involuntary movements that may occur in patients with Parkinson disease as a "complication" of long-term treatment with dopamine-enhancing medications, especially levodopa. The reason for the quotes in "complication" is that the drugs in question cannot be considered the exclusive cause of the dyskinesia. For example, persons who receive such medications for reasons other than Parkinson disease do not develop such movements. Also, it appears that a certain degree of progression of Parkinson's is necessary for dyskinesia to appear. There is an association between the total amount of levodopa a person has received, the duration of such treatment, and the likelihood of dyskinesia. However, it is not clear that this represents a cause-and-effect relationship. It may simply mean that patients with more severe forms of the disease are more prone to develop dyskinesia, but because their disease is more severe they are also more likely to have received high amounts of levodopa. Another observation is that patients who contract the disease at a younger age are likely to develop dyskinesia earlier; the reasons for this predilection are not understood.

Dyskinesia may take a variety of forms. The most usual form of dyskinesia is **chorea** (a Greek term meaning "dancelike movement"). Chorea may affect the arms, legs, trunk, or even the face muscles (resulting in involuntary grimacing). It may even affect respiratory muscles and result in irregular breathing or gasping. One side of the body may be more affected than the other. When mild, chorea may not be intrusive and many affected people may not even be aware of the movements. Severe chorea, however, may affect the balance or make it difficult for a person to sit still. Sometimes the movements may even cause a person to fall out of a chair. When the dyskinesia is this severe, it can cause weight loss and serious disability. At times dyskinesia may take the form of dystonia (discussed earlier) or myoclonus (discussed below) and can be painful.

Dyskinesia most often follows the timing of a person's levodopa dosing. Physicians distinguish between two patterns: peak-dose dyskinesia or diphasic dyskinesia. Peak-dose dyskinesia happens when the blood level of levodopa is at its highest, which is about 30–60 minutes after taking a dose. Diphasic dyskinesia is rarer and occurs as the plasma level rises, so usually within 10–30 minutes after taking a dose; it then disappears as the blood concentration of the drug peaks, only to reappear as the plasma level drops 90 minutes to a few hours after the dose was taken. Often patients have both varieties, and it may be difficult to determine the exact pattern, in which case the doctor may ask the patient to keep a detailed log every 30 minutes. Some clinics may even bring the patient in for a few hours and observe them through a couple of cycles of medication. Distinguishing between these types of dyskinesia is important, as the appropriate treatment is different for the two types.

As mentioned earlier, dyskinesia is often mild. Even when moderate, the dyskinesia may not cause any functional impairment or pain, and the patient may be only marginally aware of its presence. Since trying to treat the dyskinesia can have a negative impact on other motor symptoms of Parkinson disease, the doctor and patient may mutually agree not to take any special action. In recent years, physicians have tried to distinguish between "troublesome" and "non-troublesome" dyskinesia before deciding whether an intervention is necessary. Dyskinesia is considered troublesome when it interferes with eating, talking, dressing, sleeping, walking, social interaction, or thinking or when it causes embarrassment.

With peak-dose dyskinesia, the usual treatment involves lowering the amount of levodopa and complementing the lower dose with a different anti-Parkinson drug. There are some anti-Parkinson drugs that may actually improve dyskinesia. With diphasic dyskinesia the treatment usually involves modifications to the medication regimen that minimize the time that it takes for levodopa levels to rise and fall. More on the management of dyskinesia can be found in Chapters 7 and 9.

Myoclonus

Myoclonus is a type of quick, jerky, involuntary movement and is often seen as a form of dyskinesia in people living with Parkinson disease. The movements are more sudden than those of chorea. When severe, they may cause people to drop things or even lose their balance. Myoclonus is a relatively rare phenomenon and may respond to special medications, as well as the usual anti-Parkinson drugs. Sometimes myoclonus happens as a person is falling asleep. This is a normal phenomenon that is called nocturnal myoclonus, but it can be exacerbated by some anti-Parkinson medications and may be severe enough to interfere with falling asleep.

Fluctuations of Motor Response

Although not strictly a symptom of Parkinson disease, it's important to address the phenomenon of fluctuations in motor symptoms. Within a few years of starting treatment with levodopa, most people will experience such fluctuations, which may be either predictable or unpredictable. Fluctuations appear in up to 50 percent of patients within five years of starting levodopa treatment. The fluctuations are considered a form of treatment complication, similar to dyskinesia, and may coexist with dyskinesia. The simplest and earliest type of fluctuation to appear is the **wearing off** phenomenon. This means that the symptom relief provided by levodopa fades, or wears off, before the next dose is due to be taken. Usually wearing off is first noticed in the middle of the night after the last dose of the day or early the next morning. It may take the form of decreased mobility or dystonia. Soon, similar wearing off is noticed between doses during the daytime as well.

The reasons for motor fluctuations are not all that well understood, but several mechanisms may be involved. One of the most widely accepted mechanisms is the "loss of presynaptic buffer." This mechanism relates to the fact that any dopaminergic neurons remaining in the a patient's substantia nigra have the ability to take up levodopa, convert it to dopamine, and store the dopamine for later use. However, as the disease progresses, more dopamine cells die and the "dopamine storage capacity" of the substantia nigra declines. Eventually, the only available dopamine is what can be produced immediately from whatever amount of levodopa is present in the bloodstream at any given moment. After a person takes a dose of levodopa by mouth, its concentration in the blood rises quickly, peaking within 30–45 minutes, and then drops to less than half the peak within another 90 minutes or so. As the disease progresses, the drug's effect may last just one to two hours. This requires more frequent dosing of levodopa, the use of medications that prolong the presence of levodopa in the blood, or supplemental treatment with other anti-Parkinson drugs. As the disease progresses further, other factors may cause unpredictability in levodopa levels (such as the rate of its absorption from the intestines or interference with its absorption by foods that are high in protein content). Such factors can lead to unpredictable fluctuations of motor response, which are collectively called the **on/off phenomenon**. In this situation, motor dysfunction, such as dramatic slowing of movement, severe spasms, or tremor may appear quite quickly and unpredictably in relation to when the medication was taken. Dyskinesia may coexist with other "treatment complications" and appear at progressively lower doses of levodopa, eventually leading to what is referred to as the "reversal of the therapeutic window," when side effects such as dyskinesia (which usually reflects "too much" medicine) coexist with bradykinesia, rigidity, and tremors (which usually reflect "too little" medicine).

The wearing-off and on/off phenomena may also affect a person in other, less obvious ways. When the drug wears off or when the on/off phenomenon occurs, a patient may experience non-motor symptoms such as generalized pain, chest pain, anxiety, shortness of breath, a panicky feeling, sweating, or severe depression. Such symptoms are considered "non-motor fluctuations."

Chapter 4

The Non-Motor Symptoms

Although the most visible signs of Parkinson disease are motor symptoms that affect how a person performs many physical activities, such as walking, moving, swallowing, and writing, the disease may also cause many non-motor symptoms that affect the sensory, cognitive, emotional and psychiatric, and sometimes the automatic functions of the brain and body. When reading about the nonmotor symptoms discussed in this chapter, it is important to remember that people living with Parkinson disease will not necessarily experience all of them, and some patients may never experience any.

Sensory Symptoms

Sensory symptoms are those that affect a person's sense of smell, touch, taste, hearing, or vision. Let's start with **smell** and **taste**. People with Parkinson disease often experience a diminished sense of smell. Scientific research suggests that the sense of smell may start to diminish many years before a person develops the disease. In an eight-year study of 2,267 men, physicians at the Veteran's Administration Pacific Islands Health Care Center in Honolulu asked participants to identify the following items using only their sense of smell: pineapple, rose, soap, onion, turpentine, lemon, gasoline, cinnamon, banana, and chocolate. Over the subsequent years, 35 of these people (who were an average of 80 years old at the beginning of the study) developed Parkinson disease. Those who had received lower scores on the smell test were more likely to have contracted the illness.

> Loss of **smell** may be one of the earliest symptoms in Parkinson disease, sometimes preceding the onset of the disease by many years.

Many people don't realize that most of our sensory responses to food—both positive and negative—are due to our sense of smell. When we arrive home and our partner is cooking dinner, it's the smell of the simmering garlic or onions that gets us excited about the meal we'll soon eat.

> Loss of smell affects our sense of **taste** and causes decreased appreciation of flavor in foods.

Likewise, an unfamiliar smell while eating at an ethnic restaurant we haven't tried before might give us pause. In both instances, our sense of smell leads the way. When we eat food, much of what we taste is interpreted through our sense of smell. The sense of taste is actually limited to sweet, bitter, sour, and salty. So people who lose their sense of smell also lose some of their sense of taste. When this happens in Parkinson disease, it may contribute to weight loss. This is particularly in the more advanced stages of the disease, when the decreased enjoyment of food combines with a slowing in stomach motility (described later in this chapter) to produce a loss of appetite and loss of interest in eating.

Parkinson disease can affect **vision** in a variety of ways: loss of contrast sensitivity, double vision, and blurred vision. We discussed some of the vision problems that arise from impaired eye movement in Chapter 3. Parkinson's patients also quite frequently lose contrast sensitivity, which is the ability to distinguish between objects of similar colors based on their different brightnesses. This can lead to problems if a person, say, is looking for a scuffed-up brown baseball on a brown dirt infield or a red pen lying on top of a red tablecloth. Men and women with poor contrast sensitivity also have trouble seeing objects in dim light.

> **Blurred** or **double vision**, difficulty seeing in **dim light**, and loss of **depth perception** can be frequent problems for people living with Parkinson disease.

There are many reasons why people with Parkinson disease may have such problems with their vision. One possibility is a malfunction of the retina, the inner lining of the eyeball, which is made up of many layers of tissue. The retina contains highly specialized, light-sensitive cells and neurons dedicated to communicating the information from these cells to the brain. Based on that information, images are perceived, interpreted, and understood in the brain itself. Scientists have discovered dopamine-producing cells in the retina, so it's possible that some of the visual problems people with Parkinson experience are related to the dopamine-enhancing medications they take. Some anti-Parkinson drugs can also cause people to experience blurred vision, by decreasing their ability to adjust the size of the iris (the opening of the eye) to allow more or less light in and their ability to adjust the focus of the lens in the eye when looking at things close-up or far away. This can produce a result similar to an out-of-focus photo or one that is over- or underexposed.

Impaired movement of the eyes also has consequences for vision (as discussed in more detail in Chapter 3, on motor symptoms). People living with Parkinson disease may have double vision or have trouble "tracking" when they read. Problems with blurred vision can be worse for people with Parkinson disease who wear bifocals, trifocals, or progressive lenses, because one eye may look through the "far" part of the lens while the other eye is looking through the "near" part. Poor eye coordination may also lead to problems perceiving objects in a three-dimensional fashion and affect depth perception.

All this trouble with vision may lead people to misinterpret what they see. Sometimes, for example, they may see shadows in the margins of their field of vision. When such problems occur at the same time as a cognitive or thinking dysfunction or a psychiatric dysfunction, they may contribute to hallucinations. We'll discuss hallucinations and illusions in greater detail later in this chapter.

Parkinson disease does not, as a rule, affect the sense of **touch**. However, people with Parkinson disease *may* experience unusual sensations such as feeling crawling or tingling in their legs or feet. These may be the result of muscle spasms or restless legs syndrome, a separate disease that Parkinson patients seem to have a propensity to get. (We'll discuss restless legs syndrome in more detail in the sleep disorders section of this chapter.)

Parkinson disease doesn't tend to be a disease marked by physical **pain**, but pain does sometimes happen, mostly as a complication in the more advanced stages, but also as a symptom of the disease process itself in the earlier stages. In most cases, pain is caused by stiffening of the muscles. Sometimes this can lead to quite unusual and alarming sensations, such as chest or abdominal pain; one possible cause is stiffness of the chest-wall or abdominal-wall muscles. A patient who experiences such pains may need to visit a cardiologist or gastroenterologist to make sure there's nothing wrong with her or his heart, stomach, or intestines. These pains could hide other, more serious or even life-threatening diseases (such as a heart attack or stomach ulcers). Therefore, they should not be dismissed as an expected symptom of Parkinson disease without discussion with a qualified health care professional.

Rarely, Parkinson's patients may experience otherwise unexplained pain. Some experts have speculated that the neurodegenerative process of Parkinson disease can spread to a part of the brain responsible for sensing pain, causing what is known as central pain syndrome. This syndrome is similar to what happens sometimes (also rarely) to people who have experienced strokes and is usually treated with medications that have been specifically studied for the syndrome.

Cognitive Symptoms

Another big category of non-motor symptoms of Parkinson disease is **cognitive** symptoms, or symptoms that have to do with thinking. This category includes effects on attention; concentration; memory; communication using spoken and written language; the ability to make sound judgments, make decisions, solve problems, perform simple math, process new information, and detect and correct one's own mistakes; and self-awareness about one's own physical and mental condition and limitations.

> Mild **cognitive difficulties** can be present even in the earliest stages of Parkinson disease and should not be confused with dementia.

One cognitive function that is frequently affected in Parkinson disease—sometimes early in the course of the disease—is the **executive function** of the brain. Executive function includes the ability to make decisions, solve problems, and multitask. A big part of our executive function is working memory, the ability to maintain important information in our brain while we're engaged in complex tasks. For example, a healthy person is usually able to cook and read a recipe at the same time. While reading the next steps in a complex recipe, the cook can remember to stir the vegetables that are gently sautéing in the pan. However, a person with Parkinson disease may have trouble juggling these two tasks because of a lapse in working memory. As the disease progresses, patients may lose the ability to multitask, to perform activities with multiple steps, and to detect and correct their own mistakes. It might take them longer to think through problems and find solutions. All this sounds like a lot of trouble, but in the early stages of the disease, such **cognitive dysfunction** may not affect day-to-day activities in a major way, as one can compensate by slowing down—which happens anyway as a result of the disease. Patients with mentally demanding jobs may feel the cognitive impact of the disease sooner than others.

What Is Dementia, and What Does "Mild Cognitive Impairment" Mean?

Doctors use the term "dementia" to describe cognitive dysfunction of sufficient severity to cause major disruption in a person's day-to-day activities, to the point that the person cannot continue his or her job and may need help with everyday tasks such as paying bills or managing simple finances (for example, balancing a checkbook). To count as dementia, the dysfunction has to represent a decline from the individual's previous level of function, has to be persistent for a certain length of time (usually six months), and is not explained by a separate illness, the effect of a drug, or chemical poisoning. Therefore mild cognitive problems are not necessarily an indication of developing dementia. In fact, doctors sometimes use the term "mild cognitive impairment" to describe cognitive problems that are more than expected for a person's age but not sufficient for a diagnosis of dementia.

A diagnosis of dementia early in the course of Parkinson disease may in fact lead to a change of diagnosis from Parkinson to **dementia with Lewy bodies (DLB).**

The presence of such mild cognitive troubles should not be confused with **dementia**, which is a much broader loss of cognitive abilities. A person with dementia loses memory, has difficulty understanding simple statements and commands, can't communicate thoughts effectively, and loses the ability to perform simple daily activities. About one in three to one in four people with Parkinson disease develops dementia, but usually not until the later stages of the disease. People who experience dementia during the early stages of the disease are often referred to a specialist and may be found to have dementia with Lewy bodies (DLB), which is also known as Lewy body dementia or diffuse Lewy body disease. DLB and Parkinson disease have many similarities but are considered to be separate diseases. The dementia of Parkinson disease, also known as **Parkinson disease dementia (PDD),** is quite different from the dementia of Alzheimer disease. PDD results from the spreading of the disease process from the brainstem up into the brain hemispheres and out to the cortex, the outer layer of the hemispheres. The cortex is responsible for higher functions of thinking, understanding, putting our thoughts in words, doing calculations, learning, remembering, and using learned information to make sense of a current situation and to act and react appropriately. While Alzheimer's seems to affect the memory and language functions, PDD seems to preferentially affect the executive functions. Eventually the disease spreads to other areas as well, and in the very advanced stages, PDD may appear very similar to Alzheimer's. Thankfully, this advanced stage of dementia is seen infrequently in Parkinson disease.

Depression, apathy, and **anxiety** can be frequent "partners" of Parkinson disease.

Emotional and Psychiatric Problems

Not all Parkinson's patients experience emotional and psychiatric problems, but it does happen to some people. The most frequent of these conditions is **depression**, especially around the time of diagnosis. This is not necessarily a reaction to the diagnosis, but can be a consequence of the changes that occur in brain chemistry as a result of Parkinson disease. Some researchers theorize that depression in Parkinson patients is caused by lack of dopamine in the parts of the brain that deal with emotions. It is estimated that nearly one in two people with Parkinson disease experiences depression. Depression can dramatically affect a person's quality of life. People with depression feel sad most of the time, may lose their appetite, and may have trouble sleeping, despite feeling tired and sleepy all the time. When severe, depression can be life threatening. Affected individuals may feel hopeless, helpless, or even worthless. All enjoyment and happiness are gone from their life. They may feel that life is not worth living and even attempt to put an end to it. However, qualified health care professionals can treat depression successfully, and in most cases life-saving help may be just a phone call or an open conversation with a loved one away. It is therefore very important for Parkinson's patients to openly discuss emotional troubles with their doctors.

People with Parkinson disease sometimes experience a loss of interest without necessarily being depressed, a condition called **apathy**. This problem can be subtle and is sometimes difficult to detect, but it can affect a person's quality of life and interactions with family and friends. Prior to contracting Parkinson disease, a person may have been an enthusiastic baseball fan who enjoyed going to games with friends. Although he's still a fan, now that he has Parkinson disease he's less likely to call a friend to go to a game. People with apathy lose initiative and motivation; they become less active and more passive. Ask them if they are sad, and they say no.

These people still enjoy doing their pre-Parkinson activities; they just lack the motivation to initiate those activities. As a result, they end up relying on friends, family, and partners to ask them to do things. It's important to understand the difference between apathy and depression. People with apathy may appear sad to their family and friends, but they are not really experiencing emotional distress. On the other hand, people with depression experience serious emotional distress that may lead to loss of appetite, sleep impairment, and a loss of interest in activities.

People with Parkinson disease often have **anxiety** disorders. About half of Parkinson's patients are affected by anxiety disorders. Interestingly, some patients had anxiety disorders for years before developing symptoms of Parkinson. Sometimes the anxiety disorder is related to the wearing off or fluctuations of anti-Parkinson medication (see Chapter 3 for discussion of such effects on motor symptoms). In such cases, the anxiety disorder is nonspecific, which means that the feeling of anxiety is not directed toward a specific object or situation but is more of a generalized feeling that something horrible is about to happen. It's almost like going through a "mini-withdrawal" from the medication, and the associated feeling can be quite disconcerting, even frightening at times. When feelings of anxiety result from wearing off, they may be quite severe but are usually short-lived and self-limited.

Parkinson disease may also be associated with other, more specific forms of anxiety disorders, such as social phobia, an anxiety about interacting with other people, or panic disorder. People with Parkinson disease may have **agoraphobia**—a condition that causes a person to become nervous or jittery in large, empty spaces or in crowded rooms. Patients can also develop a fear of falling that may confine them to a wheelchair. This may happen after several Parkinson-related falls: instead of trying to continue walking or learning to walk with an assistive device, the person develops a fear of falling and becomes anxious about walking, despite the fact that he or she still has the physical ability to walk.

Impulsiveness is another psychological condition that some Parkinson's patients experience. It may be triggered by the chemical changes in the brain due to Parkinson disease, drugs used to treat the disease, preexisting personality traits, or a combination of all these factors. Impulsiveness can lead to excessive gambling, drinking, or shopping or something as simple as leaping up to answer the phone without thinking about one's physical limitations. Impulsiveness can be a particular problem when coupled with dementia.

Parkinson can also affect a person's **sex life**. People with the disease can experience loss of libido (sexual desire) or abnormally enhanced libido. This may have to do not only with the disease itself (that is, the loss of dopamine from the brain) but also with the medications that patients take to treat the symptoms. Not much is known about the mechanisms through which Parkinson disease affects a person's sex life and intimacy with a partner. People tend not to be open in talking about sexuality or may be embarrassed by their troubles. However, a 2004 study of 75 people found that a majority of women with Parkinson disease reported difficulties with arousal and reaching orgasm. Many women also had low sexual desire and sexual dissatisfaction. Among men living with Parkinson's, most said they had experienced erectile dysfunction and sexual dissatisfaction. Many men also reported instances of premature ejaculation and difficulties reaching orgasm. Not only the emotional but also the physical aspects of sexuality can be affected by Parkinson disease. This is discussed further later in this chapter in the section on autonomic nervous system dysfunction.

Hallucinations, illusions, delusions, and paranoia are all symptoms of **psychosis**, a term used to describe a disconnection between a person's perceptions and reality. Dopamine plays a central role in both Parkinson disease and psychosis.

Another large category of psychiatric dysfunctions in Parkinson disease is what physicians call **psychosis**, which, in short, means a distorted sense of reality. In people with psychosis, there is a disconnection between one's perception of reality and reality itself. This can take the form of **hallucinations**, as when a person sees or hears things that aren't there. It can also be manifest as **illusions**, as when a person misinterprets what she sees or hears. Or psychosis can be more complex, as in **paranoia**. A person with paranoia may have bizarre or abnormal thoughts. He may believe that he is being persecuted, is being followed, or is being cheated on by a spouse or partner when in fact nothing like that is actually happening. Such abnormal thoughts and ideas are called **delusions.**

Psychotic phenomena may be symptoms of Parkinson disease or may be caused by medication used to treat its motor symptoms. For decades, researchers have understood that dopamine plays a role in one's perception of reality. Shortly after World War II, psychiatrists began treating schizophrenia and other psychotic disorders with medications that fight dopamine in the brain. Many of the people treated in this way developed the physical symptoms of Parkinson disease, including tremors and loss of mobility. From these experiences, doctors concluded that too much dopamine in the brain can cause hallucinations, illusions, paranoia, and delusions. So when people living with Parkinson's began developing these kinds of symptoms, doctors believed that the symptoms were side effects of the dopamine-enhancing medications used to treat the disease. However, it soon became clear that some people developed these psychiatric symptoms even on very low doses of the medication. Therefore, it is now understood that the appearance of these kinds of symptoms in people with Parkinson disease is not only a result of dopamine-enhancing medication but may also be linked to the disease process itself. One major challenge that physicians and caregivers face is how to help a Parkinson's patient who is exhibiting psychotic symptoms. They are faced with a catch-22 situation: drugs used to combat the psychiatric symptoms lower dopamine levels in the brain, but when that happens, a person may experience more physical symptoms of Parkinson disease, such as a lack of mobility and increased tremors. Managing this situation requires a careful balancing of medications used to treat motor symptoms with medications used to treat psychiatric symptoms.

Sleep

Lots of people have **insomnia**: trouble falling asleep at bedtime or staying asleep throughout the night. Parkinson disease can complicate a person's sleep in several ways. Many people report difficulty falling asleep. Also, as the disease progresses, the medication used to treat Parkinson disease may not last long enough. A person may be able to fall asleep but may wake up in the middle of the night or just before dawn because of tremor, muscle stiffness, slowness of movement, or other similar physical symptoms causing discomfort. The person may have a tough time turning in bed or getting in and out of bed. Because the person can't move easily, she or he may have a difficult time getting into a relaxed position to sleep. All of these factors can contribute to a poor night's sleep.

> **Sleep disruption, excessive sleepiness,** and **specific sleep disorders** may all be part of Parkinson disease and may require different treatments. A careful review of any sleep symptoms with your health care provider will be necessary to develop the most effective treatment plan.

Another form of sleep disruption people may experience is **restless legs syndrome**. Although this syndrome exists as a separate condition outside the context of Parkinson's, people with

Parkinson disease are very prone to it. People with restless legs syndrome experience a sensation that is difficult to describe, but for many people it feels like an itching, burning, squeezing, pinching, or crawling sensation in the shins and calves. To relieve the sensation, people shake or twitch their legs, or they get out of bed and pace. These unpleasant feelings may happen when a person is sitting in a chair or car, but they seem to happen more frequently when the person is trying to fall asleep. Fortunately, the medications usually prescribed to treat the motor symptoms of Parkinson disease often help people who are experiencing restless legs syndrome. Some people who have restless legs may have a separate sleep disorder known as periodic movements of sleep. This disorder consists of jerking of the feet and legs while one is sleeping. This behavior may or may not disrupt one's sleep, but it usually affects how well one's partner sleeps.

Parkinson's patients often struggle with **REM sleep behavior disorder (RBD)**, a condition that involves hitting, punching, sleep talking, sleepwalking, or some combination of these behaviors as the person acts out dreams (which occur during REM, or rapid eye movement, sleep). The problem may be minor and infrequent or disruptive and constant. RBD may appear many years before the onset of Parkinson disease. In fact, many specialists consider RBD an early indication that a person may develop a neurodegenerative disease such as Parkinson's. In a 2008 Canadian study of 93 people with this problem, 26 participants developed a neurodegenerative disease within five years. Of those who developed a brain disease, most contracted Parkinson disease, but several people also had DLB and Alzheimer disease. More recent studies suggest that the proportion of people with RBD developing such degenerative diseases may climb to as much as 70% at 10 years for the diagnosis of the sleep disorder.

Sleep may also be interrupted because of **nocturia**, the need to urinate frequently at night. Nocturia may be caused by dysfunction of the autonomic nervous system as a result of Parkinson disease.

It can also be unrelated to Parkinson. Bladder control difficulties in Parkinson disease are discussed later in this chapter.

Instead of experiencing lack of sleep at night, some people with Parkinson disease have **hypersomnolence** (excessive sleepiness) during the day. This phenomenon may be the result of the disease, fatigue, or a side effect of medication. There are several aspects to the excessive daytime sleepiness besides just feeling sleepy and tired all day. Some people may experience sudden sleep attacks: falling asleep during regular activities without warning. These may be a side effect of dopamine agonists, a class of anti-Parkinson drugs. (These drugs are discussed in more detail in Chapter 7.) This is why doctors warn patients to avoid dangerous activities when beginning new medication, including long drives, climbing ladders, and operating machinery.

If a person is sleepy all day, every day, a doctor may recommend that the person be evaluated for obstructive **sleep apnea**, a disorder caused by partial or transient complete blocking of the airway while sleeping. A person with this condition actually stops breathing momentarily—sometimes for as long as 60 seconds—before waking up to take a breath, then resuming sleep. Sometimes but not always this may cause loud snoring. These awakenings may happen very frequently (up to hundreds of times in a single night), so that the person never gets deep, restful sleep. Patients may not be aware of how bad the problem is, as they do not recall waking up so many times. (To remember that we woke up, we have to be awake for longer than 10 seconds, which doesn't necessarily happen in sleep apnea.) The patient wakes up just long enough to resume breathing and then falls asleep. That's why diagnosing this condition often requires the patient to spend a night in a sleep lab. At the lab, the patient's respiration, brain waves, and blood oxygen level are continuously monitored. Anyone can be affected with sleep apnea, but overweight persons are more prone to it. Sleep apnea does not seem to be more frequent among persons living with Parkinson disease than among other people; however,

Parkinson's patients may develop sleep apnea even if they are not overweight.

Autonomic Nervous System Dysfunction

The body's autonomic nervous system controls blood pressure, body temperature, heart rate, respiration, movements of the gastrointestinal tract (the stomach and intestines), bladder movements, sweating, saliva production, and other functions that do not require voluntary control. The function of the autonomic nervous system can be impaired both by Parkinson disease and by side effects of anti-Parkinson drugs.

Orthostatic Hypotension

Orthostatic hypotension, one of the most frequent problems with autonomic dysfunction, is a dramatic drop in blood pressure when a person stands up. In its milder forms, orthostatic hypotension is experienced as a "head rush" or "dizzy spell." When functioning properly, the autonomic nervous system regulates the tone of smooth muscles inside the walls of the leg veins so that when standing, a person's blood does not pool in the legs. When blood pools in the legs, blood pressure drops, not enough blood makes it to the brain, and the person faints. Because of autonomic nervous system controls, our blood pressure stays the same whether we are lying, sitting, or standing. These mechanisms don't work as quickly in people with Parkinson disease. In addition, anti-Parkinson drugs and drugs used to treat some psychiatric symptoms of the disease may also delay or dampen the quick reaction of the autonomic nervous system. In the moderate and advanced stages of the disease, a person with Parkinson's may experience frequent or severe dizzy spells when standing up. He or she may also faint. This is more likely to happen first thing in the morning, when a person rises from bed; after a big meal; or during urination. It's not unusual for elderly men with Parkinson disease to pass out while urinating in the middle of the night. This is called micturition syncope. One way to avoid this is for the man to urinate in a sitting position.

> Because Parkinson disease affects the autonomic nervous system, it can impinge on many functions of the body not related to the ability to move. It is easy to not realize that **symptoms of autonomic dysfunction** are the result of Parkinson's, so opportunities for appropriate, effective treatment may be missed unless patients bring these symptoms up with their doctors or unless the doctors specifically ask about them.

Gastrointestinal Troubles, Nausea, and Excessive Salivation

Patients with Parkinson's frequently have constipation, both because of the disease and because of the effects of anti-Parkinson drugs on the autonomic nervous system. Constipation happens when there is a slowing down of the motions of the bowels. A similar slowing down happens with the movement of the stomach. When food stays in the stomach too long, which is called delayed gastric emptying, it can affect a person's food consumption. Although a person is hungry at the start of the meal, she or he may "fill up" quickly as a result of this condition. This can lead to loss of appetite, nausea, and weight loss. Anti-Parkinson drugs can also cause nausea. These drugs work by adding dopamine to the brain, which helps alleviate the motor symptoms of the disease. However, dopamine may trigger nausea by acting in some areas of the brain that are outside the blood–brain barrier. In fact, many nausea medications work by fighting dopamine. Such nausea medications should not be used in people with Parkinson's.

Excessive salivation is a frequent—and sometimes early—symptom of Parkinson disease. This is a complex problem that results from the combined effects of the disease process on the person's movements as a whole and on the autonomic nervous system's control of saliva production and consistency. There seems to be a true increase in the amount of saliva produced by the salivary glands of Parkinson's patients. And since the disease also causes a decline in the automatic swallowing of saliva, the combined result can be disruptive and embarrassing drooling. Treatments may not always be effective,and may cause dry mouth, a symptom sometimes worse than the drooling the treatment is meant to correct.

Bladder and Sexual Dysfunction

In addition to the change in bowel movements, bladder emptying may be a problem for people living with Parkinson disease. Most patients with bladder dysfunction have a condition called **neurogenic bladder**—also known as an overactive bladder—that causes them to go to the bathroom frequently. When combined with slowness in bladder movement, neurogenic bladder can lead to what is called overflow incontinence or urgency combined with incontinence. Several medications can be prescribed to treat this condition, although not always with excellent results. In addition, many elderly people may have other causes of bladder dysfunction, such as an enlarged prostate (in men) or stress incontinence (in women). For these reasons, doctors often may refer patients to an urologist for an evaluation. Failure of the autonomic nervous system can also cause sexual problems, such as erectile dysfunction in men and vaginal dryness and discomfort in women. More research is needed in this area, because available treatments for bladder dysfunction and sexual dysfunction don't always offer satisfactory results.

Thermoregulation

When a person feels chilly in a warm house or sweats in a cool house, the autonomic nervous system may not be regulating body temperature properly. The process of maintaining the body's temperature is called thermoregulation and may be impaired in Parkinson disease. Hot flushes, sweating episodes, or the chills may happen at any stage of the disease but are most often associated with fluctuating response to anti-Parkinson medications. Abrupt discontinuation of anti-Parkinson drugs may rarely cause a life-threatening condition, caused by a failure of the thermoregulatory mechanism, called the neuroleptic malignant syndrome. In this condition, the muscles become extremely rigid, the body temperature rises abruptly, and there may be a breakdown of muscle fibers, which can result in large amounts of protein "plugging up" the kidneys and causing serious kidney damage. The very high body temperature may also cause permanent brain damage. Although this is a very rare phenomenon, it highlights the importance of discussing any changes in the medication regimen with a qualified health care provider.

Fatigue

When a person feels exhausted without having worked, exercised, or run errands, he or she may be experiencing fatigue. This is a separate symptom from sleepiness, although the two may very well be present at the same time. Parkinson disease causes loss of muscle strength and, in some people, low blood pressure, and these symptoms can contribute to a sense of fatigue throughout the day. Fatigue also can be due to a loss of deep sleep or a side effect of anti-Parkinson drugs. There are also many other possible reasons for fatigue besides the disease itself, such as low plasma levels of certain vitamins, or hormonal problems. Increasingly, physicians are recognizing that fatigue can be a symptom of the disease, and often, but not always, a careful interview and examination may lead to the root cause and to appropriate treatment.

Skin Problems

Very early in the history of Parkinson disease, doctors realized that Parkinson patients had a tendency to have oily, flaky skin around the eyes, the nose, and the scalp. In fact, one of the earliest scales that doctors used to measure severity of Parkinson's symptoms, the Webster scale, included an item on assessing skin oiliness. This condition is called seborrhea, or seborrheic dermatitis, and is not exclusive to Parkinson's patients. Treatments vary, but severe cases ought to be referred to a dermatologist.

People with Parkinson disease may also be at elevated risk for melanoma. Melanoma is an aggressive form of skin cancer that, if untreated, can spread throughout the body and be life threatening. It stems from the melanocytes, specialized cells in our skin and mucosa (the lining of our inner cavities) that contain a pigment called melanin. Melanocytes are responsible for people's getting a tan after exposure to sunlight. Since melanin is built from molecules of dopamine, experts have wondered if there is an association between Parkinson disease, anti-Parkinson drugs, and the risk of melanoma. A few years ago, a very large and well-designed study demonstrated that Parkinson's patients have an overall higher risk of melanoma than people who do not have the disease. However, in many cases the melanoma preceded the diagnosis of Parkinson by many years and was not associated with any use of anti-Parkinson drugs. Therefore the scientists who conducted the study concluded that for reasons as yet unknown, Parkinson patients have a higher risk of developing melanoma and that the risk is not influenced by the use of anti-Parkinson drugs. This observation, however, highlights the importance for people with Parkinson disease of having regular physicals and even dermatology consultations.

Chapter 5

Diagnosis

Barrett was diagnosed with Parkinson disease at age 31. Arlene was diagnosed at age 46. Both had been experiencing tremors for a couple of years. Barrett's right hand shook occasionally. Arlene's left arm shook most of the time. Although both Barrett and Arlene experienced tremor—a common early symptom of Parkinson disease—diagnosing them with the disease had to wait till they experienced further motor symptoms. There is no single laboratory test a doctor can order to confirm whether a person has Parkinson's.

Making and Verifying the Diagnosis

When assessing a person with Parkinson-like symptoms, a physician is likely to focus on the person's medical and personal history and to perform an examination, looking for specific clues that will either confirm or disprove the diagnosis. A diagnosis of Parkinson disease is often made by a primary care physician such as an internist or a family practice physician. Since Parkinson disease is studied in detail in medical schools, most physicians can recognize the symptoms of the disease fairly readily based on the findings in the examination. However, other diseases may masquerade as Parkinson disease, so the primary care physician may refer the patient to a neurologist. To make, confirm, or reject the diagnosis, the neurologist will rely on the history that he or she receives from the patient and the patient's family and on the findings of a detailed neurological examination. Neurologists apply certain criteria in establishing a diagnosis. Different neurologists may use different sets of criteria. For the most part, the neurologist will want to see at least two of the four cardinal symptoms of the disease: tremor at rest, bradykinesia (slowness of movement), rigidity (muscle stiffness), or balance difficulties. The most strict criteria require that bradykinesia be one of the two necessary symptoms.

In addition to the typical history and findings for Parkinson's, the examining physician may also look for something called "pertinent negatives." This is medical jargon for symptoms and findings that would not be typical for early Parkinson disease. On discovering any of these items, the physician may want to reevaluate the diagnosis and proceed with additional tests to look for a different cause for the symptoms. A lot of neurologists refer to these atypical symptoms and findings as "red flags." Such red flags may lead to the diagnosis of "atypical parkinsonism," or **atypical parkinsonian syndrome**. This is a collective term doctors use to describe a group of brain diseases that share common features and may look very similar to Parkinson disease.

One such unusual symptom would be extreme balance difficulties with multiple falls during the early stages of the disease. Excessive falling in the early stages may lead to a diagnosis of **progressive supranuclear palsy (PSP)**, one such atypical parkinsonian syndrome. Of course, the physician needs to use good clinical judgment, because approximately 25 percent of all people over the age of 65 may experience repeated falls. If the falls are unexplained, clearly beyond what one would normally expect for the affected person's age, and happen early in the course of the disease, then the correct diagnosis may be one of the atypical parkinsonian syndromes rather than Parkinson's.

Another red flag is severe autonomic dysfunction in the early stages of the disease. Severe autonomic dysfunction is evident when a person shows severe and unexplained drops in blood pressure upon rising (which may lead to fainting), loses the ability to sweat in hot weather, or cannot control bladder and bowel functions (incontinence). Although such symptoms can be seen in advanced stages of Parkinson disease, they are unusual in the early stages and, if present too soon, may indicate a different diagnosis, such as **multiple systems atrophy.**

Dementia or hallucinations are not usually present when Parkinson disease is first diagnosed. If these symptoms occur in the early stages, particularly before medications have been started, a physician may consider another diagnosis, such as dementia with Lewy bodies.

In Parkinson disease it is unusual for symptoms (such as tremor) to affect both sides of the body in a very similar fashion or for the symptoms to affect the midline (like the trunk or the neck) more than the extremities (like the forearm or the foot muscles). One side is usually more affected by the disease, especially early in the disease process. If both sides are equally affected, the physician again may diagnose an atypical parkinsonian syndrome.

Similarly, severe freezing of gait early in the course of the disease—especially if combined with memory loss and complete loss of control of the bowel or the bladder—may indicate an accumulation of fluid in the brain, a condition known as **normal-pressure hydrocephalus.**

The doctor will also have to carefully review medications that the patient is taking, because some medications may cause symptoms of Parkinson's without actually causing the disease. These medications include major tranquilizers and some medications prescribed for nausea or stomach upset.

In certain situations, information from the history or findings from the examination may not disprove the diagnosis of Parkinson disease but may raise questions about whether there are any other issues to be resolved. For example, while examining a patient for Parkinson disease, a neurologist may find evidence of other, unrelated abnormalities, say, evidence of an old stroke that the patient wasn't aware of. Such a discovery may lead to additional testing, including a brain MRI scan or blood tests. In people with Parkinson disease, routine brain MRIs appear normal and therefore may not be indicated if the diagnosis is made beyond any doubt. Brain MRI abnormalities have been found in persons with Parkinson disease using specialized equipment and modified computer analysis of the MRI images. The diagnostic value of such findings is being investigated in ongoing research trials, and, therefore such testing is not as yet usable or of sufficient accuracy for general practice.

There is a lot of information available on the Internet regarding another advanced diagnostic test based on an imaging technique called positron emission tomography (PET). A PET scan can identify loss of dopamine function in the brainstem in people with Parkinson disease. If a suspected case of Parkinson disease shows no loss of dopamine, then one can safely exclude Parkinson disease as the cause of the symptoms. On the other hand, if the PET scan shows dopamine loss, that doesn't necessarily mean a person has Parkinson disease. She or he may have any number of atypical parkinsonian syndromes. Therefore a negative result is significant, but a positive result does not help a diagnosis any more than the specialist's assessment already does.

More recently another type of a brain scan, called a dopamine transporter (DAT) scan, has been approved for diagnostic use in Parkinson disease. As with a PET scan, a negative result on a DAT scan can be useful in ruling out Parkinson's, but an inconclusive or even positive result still leaves the doctor with a list of diagnostic possibilities rather than with a definite diagnosis of Parkinson disease.

Because of all the intricacies of the diagnostic process (described only briefly above), it is estimated that even with a careful history and examination of the patient, the accuracy of the diagnosis of

Parkinson disease in the early stages is approximately 80–85 percent. That still leaves a 15–20 percent possibility that further progression of a patient's symptoms will show that he or she has a disease other than Parkinson's.

The Role of the Neurologist and the Medical Team

All physicians are fully qualified to make the diagnosis of Parkinson disease. However, a primary care physician may have doubts and refer the patient to a neurologist for verification of the diagnosis. If there are further questions, the patient may be assessed by a neurologist who specializes in Parkinson disease. A neurologist of this sort is called a **movement disorders specialist**. The neurologist and the movement disorders specialist will perform a detailed neurological examination: they will examine a person's muscle tone, movements, muscle strength, reflexes, coordination, balance, and sensory system function. These doctors may also examine the person's blood pressure in reclining or sitting position and in standing position, and they may perform a brief cognitive evaluation (examination of memory and thinking).

Management of the symptoms early in the course of the disease is generally straightforward whether or not the patient is on medication. During the early stages of Parkinson disease, patients may decide to see their primary care physician more frequently than their neurologist. As Parkinson's progresses, disease management becomes more complicated, and more frequent visits to the neurologist may be required. In the moderate to advanced stages, very frequent visits may be required to readjust the treatment regimen but also to manage the increasing complexity of the multiple symptoms that emerge in time.

In the first few visits, the doctor (either the neurologist or the primary care physician) will spend time with the patient trying to explain the disease, the rationale for each treatment, and the prognosis and reviewing healthy life choices and the significance of exercise. A physical therapist may review the patient's exercise regimen and may make very specific recommendations. An occupational therapist may provide tips and ideas about how to deal with issues related to daily activities, such as how to get up from a low chair, how to get in and out of a car, how to improve mobility in bed, and how to improve one's handwriting. A speech therapist may become involved if the patient has experienced dysphonia (weakening of the voice), dysarthria (slurred speech), or dysphagia (difficulty swallowing or choking). A speech therapist may also help a patient better understand a drooling problem and how to manage it. If a patient has a partner or close relative, it is generally recommended that that person also be involved in learning about the disease, so that he or she can provide support and help to the patient now and in the future.

Many patients wonder whether doctors recommend genetic testing for Parkinson disease. There are several genes that are now known to cause Parkinson disease. Tests are available for some of these genes, but for many there are no commercially available tests. Therefore patients can obtain only a partial answer as to whether they have an abnormal type of one particular gene. Moreover, a negative test does not exclude the possibility that the person harbors some other, as yet unknown gene that causes Parkinson's. We currently know of at least 11 genes that can cause Parkinson disease, but many more are suspected. As of this writing, it is not recommended that genetic testing be undertaken for Parkinson disease with the exception of very particular cases and for research purposes. The neurologist or the movement disorders specialist will help a patient decide whether genetic testing is appropriate and if so may refer the person for further genetic counseling. (Chapter 2 discusses the genetics of Parkinson disease in more detail.)

Ask the Experts: Should I Have Genetic Testing for Parkinson's?

Dr. Martha Nance says: "Although research has shown us that genetics can play a role in determining who gets Parkinson disease, widespread genetic testing for Parkinson disease is not ready for clinics yet.

"Rare families have been identified in which Parkinson disease clearly 'runs' in the family and is directly caused by a specific gene mutation. A person who comes from such a family, where there have been multiple people over several generations with Parkinson disease, might want to discuss the possibility of genetic testing.

"Children or young adults (under age 30) who develop Parkinson disease are sometimes found to carry a mutation in one or both copies of a specific gene called Parkin*. These individuals might want to have a blood test to analyze the Parkin gene, as it might help them understand why they developed Parkinson's at such a young age. It may also clarify whether other relatives (such as siblings or children) have a higher risk of developing Parkinson disease. At this time, however, the treatment of Parkinson will not be any different if the person is known to carry a mutation in Parkin (or any other Parkinson-related gene).*

"Researchers believe that certain genetic 'variants' (changes in the DNA sequence that do not by themselves cause a disease) may increase the chance that a person will develop Parkinson disease, without directly causing the disease. Genes that may be important include LRRK-2, Parkin, and beta-glucocerebrosidase, among others. However, it is not clear which genetic variants in these genes increase the risk of Parkinson's, how much the risk is increased, and whether the risk is different in people of different ethnic backgrounds. Therefore, for the average 65- or 70-year-old person who is receiving a diagnosis of Parkinson disease and who

(Continued)

(Continued)

perhaps had a parent or cousin who also had Parkinson disease, genetic testing is not helpful.

"Another factor to consider is the cost of genetic testing. Insurers often do not pay for gene tests. And while some types of gene tests are relatively inexpensive ('targeted mutation analysis' usually costs under $500), other gene tests (sequence analysis) may cost $2,000 or more. What type of gene test a person should have depends on a detailed understanding of the particular gene and what kinds of mutations in the gene have been found in people with the disease.

"The interpretation of gene tests can also be difficult. Sometimes a patient is found to have a genetic variant that has never been seen before, and neither the laboratory nor the doctor can say for sure whether or not that gene variant is related to the disease.

"For all these reasons, genetic testing for Parkinson disease is not yet ready for routine use. In certain specific families, or for individuals from certain ethnic or geographic locations, it might be helpful. Prenatal testing or 'predictive testing' (testing of healthy individuals who have a relative with Parkinson disease) is not recommended, except in very unusual circumstances.

"Researchers continue to study the genetic aspects of Parkinson disease, so these answers may change as we learn more. Many Parkinson families have participated in these research studies, which cannot be successful without their support."

Frequently Asked Questions Regarding Diagnosis and Assembling a Team of Experts

Q: *How do I go about choosing the right physician to manage my care?*
A: Finding a physician is an important first step in your care. Although your symptoms may be first recognized and treated while

you are visiting your primary physician, eventually you may need to consult with a neurologist. A movement disorders specialist is a neurologist who has had specialized training in treating Parkinson disease and related conditions. Your primary physician may be able to recommend such a specialist, or you can seek out physicians who specialize in Parkinson's by searching Web sites of regional or national professional associations or organizations of Parkinson disease patients. (Many such organizations are listed in Chapter 13.) Attending a local educational conference on Parkinson disease may also provide insight into which physicians are involved in the local Parkinson's community.

Building a trusting relationship with your doctor will help you to cope with the disease. The doctor you work with should be willing to answer your questions and to take time to explain your symptoms and recommended treatments for your care. Make sure you feel comfortable with the physician's recommendations and that you fully understand prescribed medication schedules and potential side effects. Also be sure your physician outlines a process for how any questions or problems will be handled between appointments and that the physician shares appropriate contact information with you.

Q: Should I see other health care professionals in addition to my physician?
A: In addition to establishing a trusting relationship with a physician who fully knows and understands current trends in treating Parkinson disease, it's important to learn about the availability of other professionals who can be helpful. Ideally, these individuals will work closely with your physician to form a health care team offering integrated care focused on maximizing options for taking care of your mind, body, and spirit.

The members of your health care team will vary depending on your specific needs and the availability of various professionals in your community. Some of the team members' services will be covered by insurance, while others may not. Taking time to learn about resources in your area will help you make good decisions about seeking appropriate individuals who can provide assistance and support when needed. Your physician is a good source from which to begin learning about what resources are in the area, or you can seek advice from a local Parkinson's organization or support group. Your team may include any of the following professionals:

- **Nurse, nurse-practitioner, or physician's assistant:** A nurse often works closely with your physician and can be an excellent source for education. A nurse can also provide direction when you are seeking other health care professionals (such as therapists or social workers) to help you with specific needs. The nurse is often the primary contact person at your clinic and can help you solve problems in person and on the phone. You may also work with a nurse-practitioner or a physician's assistant on your team. Nurse-practitioners and physician's assistants are professionals with additional training that allows them to perform more detailed evaluations than nurses and to write prescriptions for medications.
- **Occupational therapist:** Previously simple tasks of daily living can sometimes become more demanding or frustrating because of Parkinson's symptoms. An occupational therapist is an excellent resource for learning ways to manage difficulties encountered at home or work. These range from techniques to improve handwriting or the use of utensils to modifications to your home or workplace that will improve safety if your balance is affected.
- **Physical therapist:** A physical therapist specializes in evaluating and treating problems associated with mobility. Physical therapy often helps patients to deal with changes in posture, walking, balance, strength, and endurance as well as other movement-related problems.

- **Speech–language pathologist:** Parkinson disease often affects communication: many people show a decrease in voice volume, produce imprecise speech, or experience changes in memory. Speech pathologists have expertise in evaluation and treatment of all aspects of communication. They also deal with issues relating to swallowing.
- **Social worker:** A social worker often provides resources and support for coping with a Parkinson's diagnosis. He or she may provide input on available services, insurance coverage, and even counsel you on how to deal with challenges in your social environment and workplace. Other mental health professionals, such as clinical **psychologists** or **psychiatrists**, may also become involved if additional counseling or medical support is needed.
- **Other therapies:** A variety of other therapists may be involved as members of your team. Music therapists, exercise physiologists, recreational therapists, art therapists, **nutritionists** (also called dietitians), chaplains and other professionals can lend support in areas of mobility, nutrition, stress management, and spiritual care.
- **Complementary medicine:** Some individuals diagnosed with Parkinson's choose to seek treatment options from alternative or complementary medicine in addition to traditional medical care. Treatments like massage, acupuncture, and naturopathy are only a few of many complementary therapy options.

Q: Is there a benefit to begin working with a team in early stages of the disease?

A: Yes. Interaction with some team members is likely to be beneficial even in early stages of Parkinson disease. Although your symptoms may be minimal, it is helpful to learn strategies that emphasize wellness and might minimize or even prevent problems in the future. Some of the newest research suggests that exercise may have a **neuroprotective** effect on the brain, helping to slow brain-cell degeneration and maximize the efficiency of remaining dopamine in the brain. Newer techniques used by rehabilitation therapists (physical, occupational, and speech experts) have been designed to capitalize on the implications of these findings by having patients work on producing large, exaggerated movements and louder voices in an effort to enhance and maintain maximal motor function. It appears that these techniques are often most effective in early stages of Parkinson disease, and the hope is that a person with early gains will be able to maintain them for longer. It is encouraged to begin other wellness strategies focusing on optimizing general health through nutrition, exercise, and stress management as soon as possible for maximal effect. Preparing for the future through advance health care directives and financial planning often offers peace of mind to people with Parkinson disease and their families.

Q: How will I work with my team on an ongoing basis?
A: Members of your team should be willing and available to answer your questions and respond to your concerns at all stages of the disease. This does not mean you will meet with every team member frequently or on an ongoing basis. You may see some team members only once or twice, while others will be involved in your care at more regular intervals. It is often helpful to become familiar with team roles early in your diagnosis, so that you have a good idea of what professionals may be most helpful in responding to a new concern. Remember that some team members will need to have a referral from your physician for their services to be covered by your medical insurance.

Q: What should I look for when seeking out professionals for my team?
A: Just as when seeking a physician for your Parkinson's care, it is helpful to ask questions regarding a potential team member's interest, experience, and training in working with Parkinson's patients. Team members should be able to clearly outline their care plans along with any associated benefits or risks of treatment. Therapists

should follow standardized practice guidelines of their professional organizations or associations and should be willing to provide you with information and answers to your questions or at least to direct you to another professional who will. Any team member should be clear about expected fees and whether her or his work is likely to be covered by medical insurance. It is often helpful to know how team members communicate with one another to ensure comprehensive and integrated care.

Q: What is my role on the team as a person with Parkinson disease?
A: Your role is the most important on a well-integrated team. It is important that your viewpoint be expressed and heard as plans for your care are developed. Make sure you are clearly defining your expectations and are working with your team by providing clear and accurate information about your symptoms and reactions to treatment. It may be helpful to write down questions or problems you are experiencing for discussion before going to appointments. Ask for clarifications if you do not understand instructions, and make every effort to follow through with recommendations for care, notifying the appropriate person if problems or questions arise.

Q: Should my family or friends be part of my team?
A: Although you will undoubtedly come into contact with a number of new individuals and professionals as you form your comprehensive care team, the people who know you best and love you most are also important members of your team. These are the people with whom you spend most of your time and on whom you rely for daily interaction and support. They may be most acutely aware of your needs and concerns and can provide important insight through their observations. You may wish to involve only one trusted care partner (partner, spouse, adult child, or friend) in your interactions with other team members, or you may wish to have more people involved. In any case, it's wise to bring someone with you

to appointments. This person can serve as another set of "listening ears," take notes, and allow you to fully interact with the team member you are visiting. It is helpful to have these individuals learn about Parkinson's through participation in appointments, classes, or educational conferences.

Chapter 6

How Will My Life Change?

Being diagnosed with a chronic illness is frightening. It's natural to focus on how Parkinson disease will make life worse. Undoubtedly life will present a person living with Parkinson's with many challenges every step of the way, and feelings of despair, disappointment, loss, and being overwhelmed may often darken one's perception of life. Nevertheless, while it seems almost impossible to believe that this unwanted life change could have any positive impact, some people have risen to this challenge, gaining insights and experiencing positive life changes. A relationship with one's partner or spouse may be strengthened. People who stop working earlier than planned may discover time for family, hobbies, and other activities. While being realistic about one's own expectations, strengths, and limitations becomes an essential part of continuing to live a balanced and rewarding life following a diagnosis of Parkinson disease, there are silver linings, and it is never wrong to try to focus on the positives.

This is one person's story:

As a teenager, Tina dreamed of becoming a painter. But she put that dream on hold for decades, working instead as a human resources manager at a small company. She married, had children, worked, and led a satisfying life.

At age 48, Tina began experiencing a slight tremor in her left hand. Other members of her family had had Parkinson disease; she was worried she might have it too. Like many other people, she preferred to ignore this warning sign, hoping it would go away. As time passed, her walking slowed and so did her arm swing. When it was apparent that things weren't getting better, Tina finally visited a doctor and was diagnosed with Parkinson disease. Despite being prepared for this particular diagnosis, the news devastated her. She worried about not being able to work and the impact a job loss might have on her family.

In the beginning, Tina wasn't experiencing symptoms that interfered with her ability to work. But as the economy slumped and people lost their jobs, Tina worried about losing her job and wondered if she'd find another one. She discussed her concerns with her boss, who was very supportive and understanding. For a few years, things were OK: medication helped ease Tina's tremor at home and work, and she was able to handle her workload. Eventually though, she lost the ability to multitask and she fell behind at work. It was taking her longer to assess problems and recommend solutions. She had another meeting with a supervisor, and accommodations were made, but Tina clearly could not keep up with the demands of her job. She was now 55 years old.

Tina also noticed that her anti-Parkinson medications were not quite as effective as when she first started taking them: there were more side effects as the dosage had to be increased, and she was experiencing more fatigue and even sleepiness. She talked to her doctor about going on disability. She felt bad about it, as she had always been a conscientious worker and also because she thought that other people could not see how truly incapacitated she was because her difficulties were not so much visible as experienced.

After a detailed discussion of her on-the-job tasks with her doctor, Tina began to think more seriously about quitting her job and going on disability. Her doctor helped her identify some tasks the disease prevented her from performing as well as additional difficulties she might encounter later on. The decision to keep working or go on disability proved difficult. Tina liked her job and she liked the people she worked with. She believed she still had a lot to offer the world and was also worried about living on less money. Still, she decided that quitting her job and going on disability was the best option.

Not working at a job gave Tina more free time. She joined an exercise class and began eating healthier foods. And she picked up the paintbrush again. Painting was a joyful, creative experience. People liked her paintings, so she began donating them to silent-auction fund-raisers for a local hospital. The paintings fetched high prices. So she painted more—and donated more.

By age 60, Tina began having increasing problems as the Parkinson's progressed. She moved slower, she experienced increased tremors, the effects of drugs began "wearing off," and she often felt tired. She still could not multitask and would never be able to go back to a "normal" job. Tina looked back at what she had accomplished and how her life had changed dramatically because of Parkinson disease. She painted frequently now, and others recognized her talent, purchasing her paintings at fund-raisers and galleries. At 60 years of age and with moderately advanced Parkinson disease, she had achieved her goal of becoming an artist. Once again, her life had meaning. One day, she wondered aloud whether her Parkinson disease was a blessing in disguise.

Although Tina's story is moving, a diagnosis of Parkinson disease does not always come with a silver lining. Parkinson's dramatically changes one's life, but no one can predict whether the change will bring some good along with the bad.

On receiving a diagnosis of Parkinson disease, one of the first questions most people ask is "What will the future look like? Will the disease sap the joy from my life?" One thing we do know is that Parkinson disease is a chronic and progressive illness. Symptoms and rates of progression vary significantly from one person to another, and there is no straightforward way of predicting one's course with the disease. Your doctor and other health care providers will not know whether you wish to learn more or will feel more comfortable knowing less about what the future holds. That's why you should openly share your fears and concerns with your physician and other members of your health care team.

Most people have a slow progression of symptoms but still will experience greater challenges as time goes on. To that end, it is important to make realistic plans for the future. Dreams that one may have had for retirement, travel, or one's financial circumstances may need to be reexamined and altered accordingly. It is important to do some soul-searching and look for ways to maintain resiliency and hope as you face this new challenge. No one can see into the future, and none of us knows what each new day will bring. Maintaining open and honest communication with your spouse or partner and trusted friends will help you share your fears, dreams, and plans. A counselor or mental health professional may offer support and assistance in coping with the fear of the unknown. Many people may turn to their spirituality to deal with these feelings and may find comfort and support in conversation with a clergy member, chaplain, or other spiritual adviser.

Reacting to the Diagnosis

A new diagnosis of Parkinson can be simply overwhelming. Each person reacts to the news in his or her own way. Many people are swept away in a sea of emotions, which may include disbelief, anger, sadness, and denial. Some people have compared receiving the diagnosis to landing unexpectedly in an isolated foreign country with no road maps or knowledge of the language or customs of the area. Others have experienced undiagnosed symptoms for some time and feel that finally receiving a diagnosis is in some way a relief. All of these emotions are normal reactions to the diagnosis of a chronic illness.

So where does one go after being diagnosed with Parkinson disease? It is natural to go through a grieving process. Many people turn to family, friends, and church, synagogue, mosque, or other house of worship for support. Sooner rather than later, most people find the strength to go on.

Seeking More Information

A second thing that happens is a desire to know more about the "enemy." Recently diagnosed people do need to learn more about Parkinson disease. Scientific studies show that patients who are better educated about the disease respond better to treatments and manage their symptoms more effectively, both in the near future and the long term. There is an abundance of information available online. Much of it may be of dubious value, but a lot of it is very useful and informative. Learning more about Parkinson disease from books such as this or from reliable sources of information such as those listed in Chapter 13 can be very helpful. It will help you understand the disease, ask the right questions of doctors, and be an informed participant in strategizing with respect to disease management.

Reviewing information that discusses every possible symptom of Parkinson disease can be distressing. It is important to know that while the disease can cause a variety of symptoms, each person is unique and experiences it differently. Avoid the tendency to compare yourself to a person you know who has or had Parkinson disease, even if that person is a parent or close relative. Symptoms, rate of progression, and response to treatment can vary significantly, especially in comparison with someone who was diagnosed many years ago, when current treatments were not available.

Shortly after diagnosis, some patients decide to get a second opinion. Often people are in denial when first diagnosed with Parkinson disease. A second opinion may be useful in clarifying any uncertainty in the diagnosis, and can be reassuring to patients and their loved ones, even if there is no doubt on the part of the diagnosing physician. As a rule, physicians are happy to provide a referral for a second opinion. Most physicians do not see a patient's request for a second opinion as an insult or as questioning their abilities. Physicians often have to deal with human suffering and insecurity, so they are generally very understanding and willing to provide such referrals on request.

Frequently Asked Questions About How to Deal with the Diagnosis of Parkinson Disease

Q: How will my life change?

A: People recently diagnosed with Parkinson disease may not notice significant changes to their daily routine. Medications frequently help most of the symptoms, and many people do not feel that their functional status has been altered. It is important for optimal health to maintain good levels of activity, obtain adequate rest, manage stress, and practice wellness strategies. Ongoing participation in leisure interests, social events, and activities that stimulate thinking and good mental health are strongly encouraged.

Some people may experience more prominent symptoms at the time of diagnosis. These symptoms should be thoroughly discussed with the physician and other members of the health care team as appropriate. Both physical symptoms and changes in mood and coping skills are of importance and may warrant further examination and treatment.

Talking to your doctor openly about your challenges in everyday activities, changes in your work abilities, and the like will help you plan better for the future and remove a lot of the stress that stems from the uncertainties of a chronic disease. While assessing what you can and cannot or should not do, it is important to focus on the positive, so that you can enrich your life in the positive areas even as you may be experiencing losses in others.

Q: How do I tell others that I have Parkinson disease?

A: It may be difficult to figure out how to go about telling your family, friends, and co-workers that you have been diagnosed with Parkinson's. There is not one "best" timetable for doing so; it is a matter of personal preference. It is sometimes helpful to first share the diagnosis with your partner or a close friend who can offer immediate emotional support. You may wish to have simple educational brochures or other resources on hand to share with people you tell of your recent diagnosis, to help them understand better what you are going through.

Remember that those you tell will also be reacting to the news and will do so in their own way. You will not have control over their responses and may find that some people need time to process the information, much as you may have when you first received the diagnosis.

Q: What does this mean for my work situation? Should I tell my employer and co-workers?

A: You are not required by law to immediately disclose your diagnosis to your employer. While some people feel comfortable sharing this information, others may be concerned that their diagnosis will affect their work relationships with their employer or colleagues. Some people find that attempting to hide the diagnosis from others escalates their stress levels and can lead to exacerbation of Parkinson disease symptoms.

It may be helpful to speak to a social worker or attorney about your rights under the Americans with Disabilities Act, which protects you and provides you with the right to request reasonable accommodations in your work environment. An occupational therapist can visit your work site and make recommendations for the accommodations that may be most helpful to you.

If you feel that your disclosure has led to a change in your work status or relationships with supervisors or colleagues, contact the company's human resources representative, seek legal representation, or do both.

If you feel that your symptoms or the medication side effects may lead to dangerous situations, however, it is important to discuss those issues both with your doctor and with your employer.

For example, if you are a long-distance truck driver and your anti-Parkinson medications make you sleepy, you need to notify your doctor, your employer, and, depending on where you live, possibly your state's transportation department.

The Next Step

The next step after receiving the diagnosis of Parkinson's will be to start dealing with the disease. You will need to make decisions such as: When should I consider taking medications? What can I do to help myself? What kinds of changes in my lifestyle will be helpful in the long term? How should I plan for the future? A lot of these questions are addressed in Chapters 7–10, on disease management.

Chapter 7

Disease Management: General Principles, Medications, and Surgery

What Are Our Weapons in Treating Parkinson Disease?

Parkinson disease is a progressive disease without a current cure. **Medications** can treat many symptoms of the disease successfully, but so far there has been little success in finding drugs that will actually slow the progression of the disease, much less cure it. Treating the symptoms, however, has allowed most patients to live longer lives. Unfortunately, the effectiveness of medications may decrease as the disease progresses, or the necessary dosages of medications may produce unacceptable complications and side effects. Some of these problems can now be addressed through a highly specialized type of brain **surgery** called deep-brain stimulation, which uses a kind of pacemaker that's inserted into the brain (more on this later in this chapter under "Brain Surgery for Parkinson Disease"). As a result of the improved medications and surgeries to treat the symptoms of Parkinson disease, patients live longer, so the disease has more time to progress. In time, these patients have to face new challenges for which existing medications and surgical treatments are inadequate. Therefore doctors and scientists are working not only toward finding a cure for the disease but also toward finding treatments for the symptoms of the more advanced stages of the disease, so that the longer lives that Parkinson's patients now have are also of better quality.

> **Medications, surgery, rehabilitation** services, **exercise**, and specialty **consultations** play complementary roles in managing the symptoms of Parkinson disease at every stage.

The challenges patients face change with every year that passes. Early in the disease, patients may experience a mild hand tremor, slight stiffness, or a lack of coordination. But as the disease progresses, other symptoms occur: a decrease of mobility, loss of balance, impaired ability to think clearly, emotional problems, and many others. For many of these symptoms, there are no drugs or surgeries that can help, so patients are taught and must learn other ways of coping with the disease. It's important that patients anticipate some of these problems and prepare for what may happen in the future. As the disease progresses, more and more health care professionals need to provide their expertise to help patients and their families along the way. These specialists may include physical therapists, occupational therapists, and speech pathologists, who can provide rehabilitation services to lessen the symptoms of the disease. Specialty consultants such as dietitians, mental health professionals, counselors, and social workers may help with several aspects of a patient's everyday life, including emotional issues and proper diet, and may assess the patient's need for assistance and provide the necessary resources. The health professionals involved in any one person's care will form this person's "team" (see also Chapter 5).

As mentioned earlier, anti-Parkinson medications are quite effective in treating most of the disease's motor symptoms, especially in the earlier stages. The decision to start medications to treat the symptoms of Parkinson disease is usually made when the person with Parkinson's and the doctor agree that the symptoms have reached a point of interfering with the person's life. If a decision is made not to start drugs immediately following the diagnosis, non-medication approaches to treating the symptoms can still be very helpful. Such approaches may include lifestyle changes, exercise, and physical, occupational, or speech therapy (depending on the types of symptoms a person experiences).

What If I Don't Want to Start Medications Right Away?

Scientific studies suggest that in early stages of the disease, some types of **exercise** may be as effective in controlling the symptoms of Parkinson disease as some of the available medications. In 2008, Dr. Victoria Goodwin of Peninsula Medical School in the United Kingdom reviewed 342 studies on the impact of exercise on Parkinson disease. Goodwin found that exercise improves physical functioning, quality of life, leg strength, balance, and walking, but the evidence was insufficient to show effects on preventing falls and the management of depression. Goodwin recommended that future research be done to establish what elements constitute optimal exercise for people with Parkinson disease.

> **Exercise** may alleviate the symptoms of Parkinson disease, and there is reason to believe that it also improves the long-term outlook for Parkinson's patients.

The effect of exercise may be more robust than the studies that have been done so far allow us to think. There are many different ways to exercise, so scientists will try to determine which types of exercise give the most benefit to people living with Parkinson disease. Although exercise can almost certainly improve some of the symptoms, no one is sure whether it also slows down the progression of the disease. Among the new symptoms patients develop with disease progression, balance problems represent a particular challenge. While there are insufficient scientific studies to show definitively that proper exercise early in the disease course can help decrease falls and other problems at later stages, many physicians and therapists who treat Parkinson disease believe this to be the case.

In a 2007 study published in the *Journal of Neuroscience*, Dr. Giselle Petzinger at the University of Southern California reported some very interesting findings. After injecting mice with MPTP—a chemical that causes Parkinson-like, dopamine-reducing damage in the brain—Petzinger examined the impact of exercise on dopamine usage in their brains. Half the mice in her experiment exercised on high-intensity treadmills, and in the other half did not. The result: Mice that exercised were faster and had better balance than the ones that did not. Petzinger also found that the dopamine-chemistry changes caused by MPTP were different in the two groups. Such evidence leads doctors to believe that besides the beneficial effect of regular exercise on Parkinson's symptoms, it may have an impact on the chemical changes inside the brains of people with Parkinson disease.

In the remainder of this chapter we will discuss medications, surgeries, and other procedures that are used to treat Parkinson disease. Chapters 8 and 10 will discuss rehabilitation, lifestyle changes, and exercise in detail. Strategies to deal with specific symptoms will be discussed in Chapter 9.

Medications

Once a decision has been made to start medications, a patient and his or her team need to decide which medication is the best.

Dopaminergic medications directly affect the dopamine chemistry in the brain in one of two ways. One is to supply the brain with levodopa—a molecule the brain can use to make dopamine. The second approach is to supply the brain with synthetic chemicals that can get in the brain and act like dopamine. These medications are called dopamine agonists. We will be examining both of these classes of medications in the next several sections.

Levodopa

Since its introduction in the 1968, levodopa (also called L-dopa) has remained the most popular and effective way to treat the symptoms of Parkinson disease. The book and the movie *Awakenings* are based on Dr. Oliver Sacks's experience with the use of levodopa when it was first introduced. Levodopa often results in dramatic improvement in the motor symptoms of Parkinson disease. However, for many patients, the effect of levodopa is not so robust. In some Parkinson patients, symptoms such as muscle stiffness and slowing improve appreciably while other symptoms, such as tremor, do not. Nevertheless, in most patients, levodopa will cause at least a noticeable improvement in most motor symptoms of Parkinson disease. In fact, when such an effect is not seen, doctors may question whether the diagnosis of Parkinson disease is correct. Levodopa was used by itself when it was first introduced, but now it is almost always used in combination with another medication. In the United States, this other medication is carbidopa.

Carbidopa is an additive that reduces the nausea caused by levodopa.

When used alone, levodopa disintegrates quickly in the liver, lungs, and kidneys. This makes it much less effective. That's why in the early years of its use its dosage had to be very high—high enough to cause severe nausea and vomiting. In the early 1970s, physicians tried to prevent this from happening by looking for a chemical that blocked the enzyme that broke down levodopa. Several such chemicals were found. Two that are in widespread use are carbidopa and benserazide. The combination of carbidopa with levodopa became widely known under the brand name Sinemet, which is a based on a combination of the Latin word "sine" (without) and the Greek word "emesis" (vomiting). So basically, Sinemet means "without vomiting." The combination of levodopa with benserazide is not available for use in the United States, but it is used widely in Europe and elsewhere in the world. Benserazide and carbidopa work in a very similar manner, so the information discussed here applies equally to both.

> The introduction of **levodopa** in the 1960s is considered one of the greatest advances in the treatment of neurologic disease of the 20th century.

The addition of carbidopa (or benserazide) to levodopa allowed a number of things to happen. The total dosage of levodopa could be dramatically reduced, because a lot more of it would make it to the brain and be converted to dopamine. Also, preventing the conversion of levodopa to dopamine outside the brain greatly reduced the nausea and vomiting caused by the levodopa when it was used alone. The combined **carbidopa/levodopa** pills come with two numbers that indicate the dosage of the medication included. For example, one formulation of carbidopa/levodopa is 25/100-milligram (mg) tablets. The first number (in this case 25) refers to milligrams of carbidopa and the second number (in this case 100) refers to milligrams of levodopa. Other formulations that are available are the 10/100-mg and 25/250-mg tablets. People who experience nausea with the 10/100 or the 25/250 tablets may do better with the 25/100 strength (more milligrams of carbidopa per milligrams of levodopa). Some people experience nausea and vomiting even with that combination of carbidopa and levodopa. To reduce nausea and vomiting, a doctor may prescribe additional carbidopa beyond what's included in the carbidopa/levodopa pills.

When levodopa was first introduced in the late 1960s, it was heralded as a miracle drug. Unfortunately, the honeymoon didn't last long. Doctors now know that most patients start to experience two undesirable side effects the longer they stay on the medication. One side effect is dyskinesia: involuntary movements such as grimacing, flailing of the arms and legs, or dancing movements of the trunk.

> **Dyskinesia** and **wearing off** may happen after a few years of treatment with levodopa.

The second undesirable effect is that although medication remains effective in controlling to a degree most of the motor symptoms of the disease, over time the duration of the effect of each dose becomes shorter. At the beginning of treatment, one can take levodopa two or three times a day and not notice any variability in the amount of symptom relief from one dose to the next. As time goes by, the effect of the medication fades (or "wears off") within a few hours of the patient's taking it. (More details about dyskinesia and wearing off can be found in Chapter 3.)

About 50 percent of patients on levodopa begin experiencing these "long-term complications" within five years of treatment. Dyskinesias and wearing off were observed for the first time in the 1970s, within the first decade of the widespread use of levodopa, and led to the suspicion that levodopa might be poisonous to the dopamine nerve cells whose function it was meant to improve. Although this theory gained momentum in the 1980s, many later studies failed to prove that levodopa is toxic. It became clear that these treatment complications weren't a result of levodopa toxicity but rather indicated a change in the way the brain handles dopamine (and levodopa) as the disease progresses. Nevertheless, the notion that delaying the use of levodopa early on will also delay the onset of complications remains strong. Some specialists dispute that notion, and there is now a trend toward using levodopa earlier in the course of the disease. New studies are being designed to assess whether using levodopa in different ways early on (for example, in small frequent or larger infrequent doses) might prevent these motor complications.

Levodopa is also associated with a number of "nuisance side effects." As has already been mentioned, some patients experience nausea. This may present quite a challenge to the physician, because antinausea medications work by blocking dopamine and therefore can easily aggravate the motor symptoms of Parkinson disease. One antinausea drug, however, can't get into the brain: domperidone alleviates the nausea of levodopa without crossing the blood–brain barrier. Domperidone is available in Canada and Europe but not the United States, because it has not been approved by the Food and Drug Administration. Another strategy to reduce the nausea caused by levodopa is to provide additional carbidopa. Carbidopa is available in the United States in a pill by itself (that is, without levodopa).

Levodopa is absorbed best on an empty stomach.

Finally, there are some tricks that patients can use to decrease the nausea-generating effect of levodopa. One such trick is to take the medication with solid foods such as crackers or bread. Another trick many people have found helpful is to use ginger. For some reason, ginger root, ginger pills, or ginger ale seem to reduce the nausea that's caused by levodopa.

However, levodopa should preferably be taken on an empty stomach. The reason for this is that levodopa is an amino acid just like the amino acids that make up proteins. When we eat something that is rich in protein, such as dairy products or meat, the proteins are broken down into amino acids in the stomach, which then are absorbed in the first part of the small intestine (the duodenum and the jejunum). However, the capacity of our body to absorb amino acids is limited, so levodopa has to compete for a "seat on the bus" with the amino acids that come from the protein in food. For this reason, doctors generally recommend that levodopa be taken on an empty stomach to maximize the amount that gets absorbed into the bloodstream. This interaction may become more important later in the course of the disease, when people start developing the wearing-off phenomenon. In the early stages it's probably OK to take levodopa with food to minimize nausea; however, most people can tolerate the drug much better after a few weeks or months, and then it is advisable to switch to taking it on an empty stomach.

Another possible side effect of levodopa (and many other anti-Parkinson medications) is confusion, and sometimes even hallucinations or paranoia. These side effects are not very frequent and happen only in the later stages of the disease. Older people are a little more vulnerable to these side effects. Just like antinausea drugs, most drugs used to treat hallucinations do so by fighting dopamine in the brain. For this reason, once hallucinations appear, a reduction in the total amount of levodopa may be necessary. Most of the time, doctors recommend other treatment modifications that we'll discuss later in this chapter under "Dopamine Agonists" and in Chapter 9.

> Both Parkinson disease and many anti-Parkinson medications may cause a **drop in blood pressure**, sometimes severe enough to cause fainting.

Levodopa may also cause a drop in blood pressure. The autonomic nervous system regulates blood pressure when we stand up by fighting the effect of gravity on blood so that when we stand up the blood doesn't pool in the feet and legs. This reflex action is dampened by levodopa, but it also is dampened by Parkinson disease itself—in both cases resulting in a sudden drop in blood pressure and fainting when a person stands up, a condition called **orthostatic hypotension**. When a patient experiences dizziness and fainting due to this condition, a doctor may recommend increasing salt intake and drinking more liquids to keep blood pressure from dropping too low, provided that the patient's heart and circulatory system are healthy. The doctor may also recommend the use of elastic stockings to prevent blood from pooling in the veins of the legs or may even prescribe medications that keep the blood pressure up by causing water retention. (Some of these medications are discussed later in this chapter under "Other Medications Used in Parkinson disease.") With a drop in blood pressure caused by anti-Parkinson medication or Parkinson's itself, patients taking drugs for high blood pressure may need to have the dosage of such antihypertensive medication adjusted, because a lower dosage may now be sufficient to control their pressure.

Finally, people with orthostatic hypotension need to be very careful about how they rise, especially when they get up from bed. They should sit at the edge of the bed and wait a moment before standing. It is generally recommended that men urinate in the sitting position, because blood pressure drops during urination. (It is not unusual for men in the more advanced stages of Parkinson disease to faint when they go to the bathroom to urinate in the middle of the night.)

There are also some precautions that one has to take when starting levodopa. The doctor has to carefully review the person's medical history. Levodopa may increase the pressure in the eye and aggravate a particular type of glaucoma. Therefore, patients with a history of glaucoma may need to have their eye pressure monitored carefully while on levodopa. Another situation in which levodopa should be used cautiously is in patients with a history of congestive heart failure. The levodopa dosage has to be increased slowly and the patient has to be watched carefully for any reemergence of symptoms of heart failure.

Carbidopa/levodopa is initially prescribed in a regimen of three times a day. The dosage may start with just half a pill three times a day and increase progressively until the symptoms are better controlled. The full effect of a dosage adjustment may not materialize until after a few (generally three to four) days. As the disease progresses, further dosage adjustments may be necessary. One adjustment is to increase the frequency with which the medication is taken throughout the day. The other is to increase or decrease the individual dose depending on the need to balance the control of symptoms against the emergence of side effects such as dyskinesias. The usual pill formulations are available in both brand name and multiple generic products but are generally colored the same way: yellow for 25/100 mg, blue for 10/100 mg, and bluish gray for 25/250 mg.

In the 1980s, a new form of carbidopa/levodopa was developed: a controlled-release formulation. Called Sinemet CR (for "controlled release"), the drug is now available in the generic form under the name carbidopa/levodopa ER (for "extended release") or SA (for "sustained action"). For simplicity we will refer to all these forms (CR, ER, SA) as ER in this chapter. This formulation is also given various names by generic manufacturers. In the earlier stages of the disease, patients can benefit from the ER version of the drug, since they need to take it only twice a day, which is more convenient than the three-times-a-day dosing of the regular formulation. Although ER formulations of levodopa have an important role in the treatment of the early and moderate stages of Parkinson disease, they do not seem as predictably effective in the more advanced stages. As the disease progresses and the long-term complications of dyskinesia and wearing off start to appear, the frequency of the ER formulation has to be increased. Under such circumstances, the effects of the ER pills may be a little less predictable than those of non-ER pills because of the less predictable absorption of the medication; at times ER pills may cause more dyskinesia and at other times more wearing off than the non-ER pills.

One area where the ER formulation has been quite helpful has been in controlling the symptoms of Parkinson disease overnight. Patients with Parkinson disease often experience slowness of movement, stiffness, and inability to get comfortable in bed at night as well as inability to fall asleep if they wake up. Some of these symptoms are improved with a bedtime dose of ER carbidopa/levodopa pills. Another useful application of the controlled-release formulations is for patients who experience nausea, headaches, or dizziness from the regular formulations of carbidopa/levodopa. These symptoms usually happen because levodopa reaches a peak in the blood plasma quickly after the medication is ingested and then the plasma level slowly drops over the next two to three hours. It is during the peak that most people experience the nuisance side effects of the medication, including nausea. With ER pills, this peak is lower and develops more slowly; the decline is also less steep. However, because the ER formulation has not really lived up to its expectations of "smoothing out" the dyskinesias and wearing off, the quest to find a formulation of levodopa that will not cause the "ups and downs" in the moderate to advanced stages of the disease continues.

In the last few years carbidopa/levodopa has become available in an orally disintegrating tablet form, under the brand name Parcopa. This pill is easier to take than other forms when there is no water readily available, such as when one has to take a pill in the middle of the workday, in a plane or a car, or even in the middle of the night.

Scientists are also working on developing a gel formulation of the medication that can be administered in a continuous fashion straight into the stomach. Studies of this latter formulation have shown that it minimizes the long-term complications of dyskinesia and wearing off.

Researchers have also focused on developing medications that extend the effectiveness of levodopa by making it last longer in a the bloodstream. Such medications block or slow down the breakdown of levodopa and dopamine. A number of such medications have been developed and are available for use. One of these medications is called entacapone and is discussed later in this chapter under "Levodopa Extenders." The company that manufactures entacapone has also produced a formulation that contains carbidopa/levodopa and entacapone in one pill.

Dopamine Agonists

Since medical experts first realized that levodopa can cause abnormal, involuntary movements in Parkinson patients, scientists have attempted to produce synthetic chemicals that would stimulate the dopamine receptors in the brain directly, thus "bypassing" dopamine. In other words, the effort concentrated on creating drugs that act in dopamine's place. These efforts resulted in several drugs that are collectively called **dopamine agonists**. Some of these medications have been successful in treating Parkinson disease, while others have been approved for other diseases where dopamine action is needed but not for Parkinson's. The so-called first generation of dopamine agonists includes bromocriptine (also known by the brand name Parlodel) and pergolide (also known by the brand name Permax). Subsequent efforts have created a second generation of dopamine agonists. These are pramipexole (also known by the brand name Mirapex) and ropinirole (also known by the brand name Requip). All four of these are in pill form. Most recently another dopamine agonist was developed that can be used in a patch form, so that the medication is absorbed through the skin rather than through the stomach. This is called rotigotine (also known by the brand name Neupro). One more dopamine agonist, apomorphine (brand name Apokyn) is available in injection form. There are other dopamine agonists used in Canada and Europe that have not been approved by the U.S. Food and Drug Administration, including piribedil and cabergoline. Pergolide has been withdrawn from circulation. After many years of use, some patients who took it developed problems with their heart valves. As a result, the company that produced pergolide voluntarily withdrew it from the U.S. market in 2007.

This leaves five dopamine agonists that are currently available for use in the United States: bromocriptine, pramipexole, ropinirole, rotigotine, and apomorphine. The first three, all pills, share certain characteristics. They all have relatively long half-lives, which means that they linger in the bloodstream for a longer time than levodopa. This is a helpful property when levodopa wears off. However, none of these medications is as potent as levodopa in controlling the symptoms of Parkinson disease, and therefore patients with Parkinson disease will sometimes continue to experience the wearing-off effect of the levodopa despite the addition of a dopamine agonist.

Another use of dopamine agonists is early on, when symptoms are relatively mild and the full potency of levodopa is not considered necessary. By using dopamine agonists, one aims to delay the need for levodopa and the occurrence of dyskinesia and wearing off. As mentioned earlier, in the discussion of levodopa, the notion that delaying use of levodopa forestalls those complications is not fully accepted by all Parkinson specialists. As a group, dopamine agonists can cause nausea and vomiting, and it's usually recommended that patients take them with food. These drugs are usually taken three times per day. Lately two of them—ropinirole and pramipexole—have become available in the United States in a time-release form that can be taken once or twice a day.

Dopamine agonists have a number of side effects in common, but they also have some individual differences. They can all cause nausea, because they stimulate dopamine receptors outside the brain as well as inside. Just like levodopa, they can cause a decrease in blood pressure and they may be associated with an increased propensity for hallucinations and paranoia. They may cause confusion, excessive daytime sleepiness, and personality and behavioral changes. Another side effect is swelling around the ankles and water retention. Not everybody who tries these medications experiences these side effects. However, there are two major side effects that patients and their families should know about in particular. These are excessive daytime sleepiness and personality and behavioral changes. Although these side effects are not always encountered, they may have very serious implications when they occur.

Excessive daytime sleepiness can be experienced either as feeling sleepy and tired throughout the day or as sudden episodes of sleep (also called sleep attacks) that happen without warning during the day. Although the latter form of excessive daytime sleepiness is extremely rare, its consequences can be deadly if the sleep attack happens while a person is driving or operating heavy machinery or in similar situations. For this reason, doctors usually ask patients not to drive or operate heavy machinery during the first few days or weeks of treatment with dopamine agonist medications, until they know how the medication affects them.

Sudden **sleep attacks** and personality changes with **obsessive, impulsive, and compulsive behaviors** are two potentially very serious side effects of dopamine agonists.

The second side effect with potentially serious consequences is personality and behavioral changes. Some patients who take dopamine agonists develop obsessive, impulsive, and compulsive behaviors. Such behaviors include excessive gambling or shopping, punding (a term that refers to obsessively taking things apart and putting them together; performing repetitive, seemingly purposeless tasks, such as sorting or rearranging various objects; or collecting trivial items), starting multiple projects and never finishing them, and obsessing about sexual matters. A reduction in dose sometimes helps with such side effects, but if that's not sufficient and the side effect is serious, then the medication should be discontinued. When some medication is absolutely necessary, a switch to another drug in the same category (that is, a different dopamine agonist) may sufficiently control the Parkinson symptoms without the side effects. If this strategy doesn't work, other medications can be used to control the abnormal behaviors (more on these medications later in this chapter under "Other Medications Used in Parkinson Disease"). If the behaviors are neither intrusive nor harmful, simple counseling of the patient and the care partner is sometimes sufficient.

Bromocriptine has one additional potentially serious side effect that may appear after long-term use. This is the development of abnormal fibrous tissue in the abdominal cavity or damage to the fingertips or toes. This complication is extremely rare, but patients and care partners need to be aware of it, so that the medication can be discontinued if such signs appear.

Pramipexole is largely cleared from the body through the kidneys. Therefore the dosage may need to be reduced in people who have kidney damage or develop kidney damage. Pramipexole itself does not cause kidney damage. In the presence of kidney damage, however, pramipexole may accumulate in the bloodstream, reaching toxic levels and causing severe side effects, including confusion, severe hallucinations, and sleepiness.

Ropinirole warrants a specific warning: This medication is metabolized (broken down) by the liver. Special enzymes produced by liver cells are responsible for breaking down not only ropinirole but also other medications and nutrients. Among the latter substances are estrogens and the antibiotic ciprofloxacin. Both of these interfere with the breakdown of ropinirole by the liver and may lead to increased side effects from the medication. This is a good example of why it is important to pay attention to any warnings and information that pharmacists supply when dispensing medications.

Rotigotine is a patch that needs to be replaced every day. It is important that the old patch is removed when the new one is applied, or an overdose may occur. A side effect particular to this medication is a skin reaction where the patch is applied, and therefore the location needs to change every day. Sometimes the skin reaction may be severe and affect areas of the body where the patch was never applied, and in this case, the medication needs to be discontinued.

In addition to Parkinson disease, dopamine agonists are used for the treatment of restless legs syndrome. Since patients with Parkinson disease are also prone to develop this syndrome, sometimes an evening or bedtime dose of a dopamine agonist is added to levodopa just to help control restless legs.

As people get older, they also become more sensitive to the cognitive and psychiatric side effects of dopamine agonists, which include confusion, hallucinations, and paranoia. Therefore quite often in the more advanced stages of the disease and especially once cognitive symptoms have appeared, doctors slowly withdraw dopamine agonists and focus on maximizing the dosage of levodopa to minimize the risk of side effects.

One dopamine agonist is almost in a category of its own. This is apomorphine hydrochloride (known under the brand name Apokyn). Unlike the pills discussed above, rhis medication does not get absorbed through the stomach but rather is administered through a subcutaneous injection. It is very fast acting, but its effect also dissipates very rapidly. Because of this, apomorphine is not used for the routine management of Parkinson disease but rather serves as a "rescue therapy" for people with advanced Parkinson disease who experience a lot of fluctuations. The term "rescue" simply refers to the fact that an injection of apomorphine may restore mobility in a person whose recent dose of levodopa has worn off and who is not due for another dose for an hour or two; apomorphine "rescues" the person from having to endure the increased symptoms until the next dose of levodopa. Because the effect of the medication is short-lived, the chance of added side effects when the patient takes the next scheduled dose of levodopa is minimized. Apomorphine has the potential for side effects similar to those of the dopamine agonists described above. Its dosage has to be fine-tuned for each patient. Initiation of treatment with apomorphine takes place in the doctor's office, because it is a fairly potent medication and can cause nausea, vomiting, and a severe drop in blood pressure. Some patients may need to take an antiemetic (antinausea) medication in combination with apomorphine injections.

Levodopa "Extenders"

> Levodopa extenders work by blocking one of two enzymes responsible for the breakdown of levodopa and dopamine; these enzymes are **MAO-B** and **COMT**.

Another strategy for improving dopamine function in the brain is to use medications that slow the breakdown of dopamine or the breakdown of levodopa. These medications act by blocking certain enzymes either in the brain or in the liver, lungs, and kidneys. Two such enzymes have been the target of these medications: monoamine oxidase type B (MAO-B) and catechol-*O*-methyltransferase (COMT). The classes of medications used to block these enzymes are respectively called **MAO-B inhibitors** and **COMT inhibitors**. There are two medications available in each class in the United

States. The MAO-B inhibitors are selegiline and rasagiline. Available COMT inhibitors are entacapone and tolcapone. These medications allow the brain dopamine to last a little longer and therefore extend the duration of the levodopa effect, sometimes by as much as 20–30 percent.

MAO-B Inhibitors

What is most interesting about MAO-B inhibitors is that scientific research suggests that they may slow the progression of Parkinson disease. This possibility was raised when scientists discovered that MAO-B was found to mediate the toxic effect of MPTP in dopamine neurons. So in the 1980s, Parkinson's researchers in the United States and Canada began a large study, known under the acronym DATATOP, to see if MAO-B inhibitors would slow the progress of the disease. In 1988 scientists reported that Parkinson disease patients who received selegiline for about two years had a more benign course of the disease and better symptom control than patients who received a placebo. The study also found that patients who received selegiline did not need to start treatment with levodopa as early as patients who received placebo.

However, the DATATOP study's conclusions were somewhat flawed. Researchers at the time had not realized that selegiline improves the symptoms of Parkinson disease for weeks *after* the medication is discontinued. As a result the study's designers had not taken this so-called symptomatic effect into account. So despite initial excitement about the DATATOP results, doctors progressively became less convinced that selegiline did indeed slow the steady march of Parkinson disease. Moreover, as selegiline was used more extensively, doctors noted that patients who received the medication experienced a number of side effects, such as confusion, hallucinations, and difficulty sleeping. Selegiline is absorbed in the stomach and goes through the liver before it reaches the brain. In the liver a portion of it is converted into amphetamine-like compounds. These amphetamine-like by-products of selegiline are blamed for the confusion, hallucinations, and insomnia. Older patients are particularly susceptible to these side effects.

To lessen the shortcomings of selegiline, researchers developed an orally absorbed form of the medication under the brand name Zelapar. Zelapar is formulated in a tablet that dissolves in and is absorbed in the mouth. It does not have to go through the liver before reaching the brain. As a result, the dosage can be decreased to as little as 1.25–2.5 mg a day, which is about one-eighth to one-quarter of the dosage of regular selegiline. By avoiding the breakdown of large quantities of selegiline in the liver, Zelapar achieves two goals: there are fewer toxic breakdown products, and most of the selegiline makes it to the brain without being lost in the liver.

The **DATATOP** and **ADAGIO** trials have suggested that MAO-B inhibitors like selegiline and rasagiline may slow down the progression of Parkinson disease; however, doubts remain, and more research is needed to prove this notion.

Another MAO-B inhibitor is rasagiline (brand name Azilect). This medication has a similar function to selegiline, but it lacks many of selegiline's toxic by-products. Like selegiline, Zelapar and rasagiline are eventually broken down in the liver. Because of this, care should be taken when Zelapar or rasagiline is given in combination with other medications that have to be processed in the liver, because interactions between the medications may occur.

It is thought that MAO-B inhibitors may cause a dangerous increase in blood pressure if taken together with certain types of antidepressants, over-the-counter medications, and narcotic analgesics. Similar interactions may occur with certain foods or beverages that are rich in the amino acid tyramine, which is found in aged and fermented cheeses, red wine, and cured and preserved meats. However, this concern about MAO-B inhibitors is based on the chemistry of these drugs and of tyramine and not on actual occurrences of blood pressure "spikes." Studies are under way to see if caution about avoiding these drugs and tyramine when taking MAO-B inhibitors is warranted. MAO-B inhibitors nevertheless come with a long list of over-the counter drugs and foods to avoid, although the list has recently been considerably shortened by the Food and Drug Administration. This list is usually supplied by the pharmacist when a prescription is filled and should be carefully consulted when a patient is starting an MAO-B inhibitor.

As soon as the less-toxic MAO-B inhibitors were available, scientists decided to investigate again their potential to slow the progression of Parkinson disease. In a 2009 study of more than 1,000 patients, called the ADAGIO trial, researchers found that rasagiline may indeed have such an effect. Study participants were treated with rasagiline or a placebo. Two doses of rasagiline were tested: 1 mg per day and 2 mg per day. This large study reached certain conclusions that may at first sight appear somewhat counterintuitive and contradictory. The investigators concluded that 1 mg a day of rasagiline did provide a **disease-modifying** effect, meaning that patients who received 1 mg of rasagiline a day gained some ground over patients who received placebo for the first six months of the study and then started rasagiline. The people who started the rasagiline earlier maintained this advantage over the late starters until the end of the study. However, this disease-modifying effect wasn't observed in patients who took 2 mg of rasagiline a day. Scientists aren't sure why this happened; however, it is known that some drugs do work better at lower doses. Further studies will be needed to determine whether rasagiline is indeed capable of slowing down the progression of Parkinson's.

In practical use, selegiline is taken in a dose of 5 mg in the morning and in the early afternoon (to avoid nighttime insomnia and nightmares). Zelapar is administered once in the morning; it is taken by mouth and is allowed to dissolve and be absorbed in the mouth. Food and drink should not be taken for a few minutes after the intake of Zelapar. The usual starting dosage is 1.25 mg, or one tablet, in the morning. After six weeks, this dosage can be increased to 2.5 mg, or two tablets, in the morning. Finally, rasagiline is given in a pill form, and the usual starting dosage is 0.5 mg in the morning, which can be increased to 1 mg in the morning. All these medications have the ability to prolong the effectiveness of levodopa by as much as 20 percent. Because they increase the available amount of dopamine in the brain, side effects may include dyskinesia, nausea, vomiting, hallucinations, and confusion. MAO-B inhibitors are often prescribed early in the disease to treat mild symptoms so as to conserve dopamine agonists and levodopa for a later time.

COMT Inhibitors

The second class of levodopa and dopamine extenders is the COMT inhibitors, which act through the enzyme catechol-O-methyltransferase. This enzyme is found in the liver, kidney, and lungs as well as in the brain. There are two medications in this category: entacapone (brand name Comtan) and tolcapone (brand name Tasmar). There is also a pill that contains carbidopa, levodopa, and entacapone. This formulation is called Stalevo. Initial studies with these medications showed that patients who experience the wearing-off phenomenon had an increase in "on" time of between 20 and 60 percent.

As with the MAO-B inhibitors, the fact that COMT inhibitors block the breakdown of levodopa and dopamine can results in several side effects, including low blood pressure, dizziness, light-headedness, nausea, vomiting, confusion, hallucinations, and sleepiness. Dyskinesia can be exaggerated by these medications. Additional side effects are particular to each of the COMT inhibitors. Both entacapone and tolcapone can cause severe diarrhea, which sometimes eases with continued use of the medication. With entacapone, saliva may turn slightly yellow, and urine may turn a dark orange-brown color. This does not happen to everyone who takes entacapone, but if it happens, it is simply the result of the way the person's liver processes the medication and is not an indication of a serious adverse reaction. It is not a reason to discontinue treatment.

Tolcapone has a potentially serious side effect. It can cause severe, irreversible liver damage that can lead to a need for a liver transplant. Although very few cases with this side effect have been reported, patients who go on tolcapone are required to review warnings of this effect and sign an agreement to receive the medication. Blood tests of liver function have to be done before the first dose and then again frequently—every two weeks—in the early months of the treatment; later on the frequency can decrease to once a month or every two months. A difference between entacapone and tolcapone is that entacapone blocks COMT mostly outside the blood–brain barrier, while tolcapone might also block COMT inside the brain. Another difference is that patients take a 200-mg dose of entacapone with every dose of levodopa, whereas tolcapone is administered three times a day at a dose ranging between 100 and 200 mg each time.

> Older medications such as **anticholinergics** and **amantadine** may be helpful in special cases; however they often have many "nuisance side effects," particularly among the elderly.

Anticholinergics and Amantadine

In this section, we will discuss medications that do not act directly on the dopamine system. Most of these medications are anticholinergic drugs. The reason for this name is that these medications work against **acetylcholine**, a neurotransmitter in the brain.

Neurotransmitters are chemicals produced in the brain that neurons use to communicate with each other. Dopamine ais also a neurotransmitter. Dopamine and acetylcholine have somewhat opposing actions on motor function, regulation of muscle tone, and the production of tremors. Early in the history of treatment of Parkinson disease, doctors thought resetting the balance between dopamine and acetylcholine in the brain might alleviate some of the motor symptoms of Parkinson's. To reset this balance, doctors used medications that suppressed the function of acetylcholine. These medications were somewhat effective and are still used today.

Unfortunately, acetylcholine has a lot of functions besides regulation of muscle tone, so anticholinergic medications often have many unwanted side effects. For example, acetylcholine is very important in memory functions. As a result, people who take medications that fight acetylcholine may occasionally experience confusion. This is especially true for older people. Acetylcholine is also a pivotal in regulating the autonomic nervous system, so people who take anticholinergics may experience blurred vision, constipation, muscle cramps, difficulty with initiating the stream when they urinate, erectile dysfunction, and sleepiness. Younger people experience fewer side effects when taking these medications, so sometimes anticholinergics are used early in the treatment of the disease, especially if delaying the use of a dopamine agonist or levodopa is desirable.

Medications in this category include trihexyphenidyl (brand name Artane) and benztropine (brand name Cogentin). Sometimes patients will be put on these medications early on and may experience a good effect in controlling motor symptoms. As the disease progresses, however, patients may start noticing more cognitive difficulties. At that point the doctor may discontinue the anticholinergic medication. In fact, anticholinergics are one of the first medications to go once a person starts to have cognitive dysfunction.

Another medication used for treatment of motor symptoms of Parkinson disease is amantadine, which is not an anticholinergic (brand name Symmetrel). Amantidine was first produced in the 1960s as an antiviral agent. It has been used and sometimes is still used for the treatment of the flu. Amantadine improves some of the symptoms of Parkinson's in some patients. Initially it was thought to be quite good for tremor, but it was later noticed that the effect on tremor may fade after a few months. Many Parkinson disease specialists prescribe it for younger patients who don't want to start levodopa early and who don't tolerate other medications well. Amantidine can cause hallucinations and confusion, especially in older people and the cognitively impaired. It is available both in a capsule form and in a liquid form and is usually given twice a day, although some patients can tolerate three or even four doses a day. One of the side effects may include swelling of the ankles and a rash called livedo reticularis, which makes one's skin look blotchy. Particularly in older patients it may cause dizziness and lightheadedness.

Over the years it was noted that sometimes patients who were taking amantadine experienced less dyskinesia than people who weren't. This led to scientific studies that found that dyskinesia responds favorably to the use of amantadine. So lately, in addition to using amantadine in the early stages of the disease, doctors have started prescribing it for dyskinesia. Although it is not a very potent medication for that purpose, some patients experience very good relief of dyskinesia. Amantadine has also been used in other neurologic diseases to alleviate fatigue, and some small studies have suggested that amantadine may be helpful in the treatment of balance difficulties. However, clinical experience suggests that in Parkinson patients such effects are generally very weak.

Other Medications Used in Parkinson Disease

As is mentioned many times throughout this book, we now understand Parkinson disease as a condition that can affect many areas of the brain beyond the dopaminergic neurons and can produce many symptoms that have nothing to do with motor function or with the dopamine levels in the brain. It follows that doctors may use medications besides the ones covered in detail above to treat these symptoms. Generally these medications are "borrowed" from other diseases and even from medical specialties other than neurology. While some of these medications have been approved for use in Parkinson's patients, many of them are used "off label" to treat the symptoms of Parkinson disease. That expression means that the Food and Drug Administration has not given approval for use of the medication specifically to treat patients with Parkinson disease. Therefore off-label medications have to be used with caution and under the close supervision of a physician with experience in treating Parkinson's patients.

It is beyond the purpose of this book to examine all these medications in great detail, especially since many Parkinson patients will never need to use most of them. It suffices here to say that whenever a new medication is introduced into your treatment regimen, you and your care partner need to understand the reason for its use, what the desired effect is, and what side effects to watch for. We will briefly describe here the classes of medications that are often employed for Parkinson symptoms that do not respond to modification of dopamine chemistry.

Medications for Tremor

Levodopa, dopamine agonists, MAO-B inhibitors, anticholinergics, and amantadine can be very effective in treating the resting tremor that is typical of Parkinson patients. However, as many as 20 percent of Parkinson patients may have a resting tremor that does not respond fully to these traditional anti-Parkinson medications. Additionally, these drugs may not be very effective for tremor that occurs with action (for example, writing or reaching for a coffee mug) or with holding something (for example, holding and reading a newspaper). Faced with such a challenge, the physician may decide to try medications used for treating a different movement disorder called essential tremor, which is characterized by action and postural tremors rather than rest tremors. These medications may include beta-blockers (a class of medications used mainly for the treatment of high blood pressure and some heart problems) or certain seizure medications. Propranolol is a representative of the beta-blockers, while primidone and topiramate are among the seizure medications.

Sometimes tremor is only an intermittent but still bothersome annoyance (for example, when it occurs in social situations and is felt to be embarrassing). In that case doctors may prescribe a mild tranquilizer, which can be used sparingly and only for problematic occasions. These medications usually are benzodiazepines, the same category as the familiar tranquilizer Valium°, and therefore should be used with caution and never be mixed with alcohol. Because they can cause or increase sleepiness, one should not drive or operate machinery when using these medications until their effects are known.

Medications for Insomnia, Excessive Daytime Sleepiness, and Other Sleep Disorders

Sometimes the reason for insomnia in Parkinson's patients is discomfort from stiff muscles or inability to get comfortable in bed because of bradykinesia. At other times tremor may keep a person up or may wake him or her up in the middle of the night when the effect of medication taken earlier in the day wears off. Restless legs syndrome is another frequent culprit. All these causes of insomnia may respond to a bedtime or middle-of-the-night dose of levodopa or a dopamine agonist. If insomnia persists despite such treatments, sleeping aids may be used. Over-the-counter sleep aids such as diphenhydramine (known under the brand name Benadryl), or the natural hormone melatonin can help. If all else fails the physician may prescribe an antidepressant that has a sedative effect, especially if depression is also a problem. Older antidepressants such as amitriptyline or trazodone can be quite effective in treating both insomnia and depression in Parkinson disease, but they may also cause a number of side effects. They therefore should be used cautiously and be started at a very low dose, tapering up depending on effectiveness and tolerability. Traditional sleeping pills can be used as well, but since most of them can lose their effectiveness with continued use or, what's worse, cause dependence (which means inability to sleep without the pill), they should be used sparingly and under close monitoring from the patient's physician.

Nightmares and REM sleep behavioral disorder respond exceptionally well to a tranquilizer called clonazepam. This medication is a benzodiazepine and therefore should be used with caution, especially since it may cause confusion in the elderly. Fortunately, low doses of clonazepam are often quite effective and are usually well tolerated.

Excessive daytime sleepiness may be a side effect of the dopamine agonists or even levodopa, and often a change in the drug regimen will fix the problem. If not, doctors may decide to prescribe medications used for narcolepsy, a condition where people may fall asleep in the middle of the day without warning. The use of such medicines has not been proven to be helpful in people with both Parkinson's and sleepiness, because there have not been sufficient clinical studies. Again, a decision for such off-label use of these medications should be accompanied by a careful review of the risks involved and the severity and disruptiveness of the symptom.

Dementia Medications

The last decade has seen a proliferation of medications for dementia, developed primarily for the treatment of Alzheimer disease. Naturally the same medications have been assessed for their effectiveness in treating Parkinson disease dementia. In fact, one of them, rivastigmine, (also known under the brand name Exelon) has been approved by the Food and Drug Administration for that purpose. Rivastigmine is available both as a capsule and as a patch. Other medications in the same category as rivastigmine include donepezil (brand name Aricept), and galantamine (brand name Razadyne). All these medications exert their action by enhancing the function of the neurotransmitter acetylcholine. Acetylcholine is to Alzheimer disease what dopamine is to Parkinson disease. As discussed earlier in this chapter, acetylcholine works against dopamine, so one might think that using medications that enhance acetylcholine in Parkinson disease might cause more motor problems. Fortunately, this has not been the case in a number of clinical studies, although there is the occasional patient in whom these drugs cause increased tremors or freezing. Some of the side effects seen with this class of medications are muscle cramping, diarrhea, worsening of stomach ulcers, nausea, worsening of irregular heartbeat, and even bad breath.

Another dementia medication, called memantine (brand name Namenda), works through a mechanism that bypasses acetylcholine. Clinical studies have shown that memantine is well tolerated by patients with Parkinson disease dementia, but there have not yet been large enough studies to assess its effectiveness.

Antipsychotics

Antipsychotics are medications used to treat hallucinations, delusions, and paranoia. The main mechanism of action of these medications is to block dopamine, and all but two have been shown to aggravate motor symptoms of Parkinson disease. The two that don't are quetiapine and clozapine. Quetiapine (brand name Seroquel) has been well tolerated by Parkinson patients in clinical studies but has been found to be at best mildly effective. It can cause sleepiness and orthostatic hypotension. Clozapine (brand name Clozaril) has been shown to be more effective than quetiapine in controlling hallucinations and paranoia in Parkinson patients but has the unfortunate risk of a life-threatening side effect: permanent and irreversible damage to the bone marrow, which may require a bone marrow transplant. Although this complication is rare, it is severe enough that it is now required that patients taking the medication have their counts of white cell bloods and neutrophils (a particular type of white cell) checked once a week while taking this medication. The frequency of testing may decrease to every two weeks after six months, and to every four weeks after the first year of treatment. As a general warning, there is evidence that elderly dementia patients treated with such antipsychotics have a higher risk of being diagnosed with diabetes and may also have a decreased life span than patients who do not need such treatment.

Medications for Orthostatic Hypotension

When the Parkinson's patient starts having trouble maintaining a high enough blood pressure when getting up, fainting may occur. The first action the doctor will take is to adjust any blood pressure medications the patient may have been taking and recommend strategies to reduce the problem, which are discussed in Chapter 9. If all else fails, however, the doctor may decide to use medications to increase the person's blood pressure. Such medications include fludrocortisone (brand name Florinef), which increases sodium and water retention; midodrine, (brand name ProAmatine), which stimulates adrenaline receptors in the veins and arteries; and even salt pills (sodium is well known to increase blood pressure). Another medication that has been found helpful in treating orthostatic hypotension is pyridostigmine (brand name Mestinon), which is used for myasthenia gravis, a condition affecting the nerve endings in the muscles. Of course any attempt to increase the blood pressure may result in increased strain on the circulation (by causing fluid overload in the case of fludrocortisone or by causing the blood pressure to be very high in the reclining position in the case of midodrine). Therefore these medications require close supervision by the patient's physician. Purchasing a blood-pressure-measuring device for home use may be necessary, so that frequent checks can be done at various times of the day and in various positions (such as in bed vs. standing up).

Botulinum Toxin Injections

Quite often changes in anti-Parkinson medications, such as adjustment of the dose of levodopa or a dopamine agonist or the addition of an anticholinergic agent or amantadine, will ameliorate dystonia. But when everything else fails, and depending on the muscles affected by the dystonia, the doctor may recommend botulinum toxin injections. Botulinum toxin is a poison produced by the bacteria that cause a severe muscle disease, called botulism, that one can catch from poorly canned foods. This toxin poisons the connection between nerves and muscles, effectively paralyzing a person's muscles. When injected in small quantities in individual muscles, botulinum toxin may alleviate the spasms of dystonia for a few months. The doctor, patient, and care partner must engage in a careful examination of the pros and cons before the decision to proceed with injection can be made. It is important to have a good understanding of what are reasonable expectations. If effective, the injections will need to be repeated every few months (usually every three or more months) because the effect is transient. The possible risks and complications vary depending on the site of the injection, the person's other medical conditions, and other medications they may be taking. In any case, too-frequent injections should be avoided, as immunity to the drug may develop. Lately botulinum toxin injections have also been approved by the Food and Drug Administration for the treatment of excessive salivation in Parkinson disease. In that case the drug is injected into the salivary glands.

Medications for Nausea

Nausea is a frequent side effect of many anti-Parkinson medications. Most of the time starting such nausea-causing drugs at a very low dose and progressively tapering up ("start low and go slow") minimizes the nausea effect. At other times, however, doctors may prescribe taking different medications with the anti-Parkinson drug to minimize nausea. One such antinausea drug is carbidopa (brand name Lodosyn), which is also a component of many pills that contain levodopa. An extra amount of carbidopa (usually 25 mg taken together with or a little earlier than each carbidopa/levodopa dose) may be sufficient to treat the nausea caused by carbidopa/levodopa. Domperidone, another nausea medication, is discussed earlier in this chapter under "Levodopa." For most people nausea stops being a problem with time. Many other nausea medications can worsen the motor symptoms of Parkinson disease and should therefore be prescribed with caution and only if absolutely necessary. Sometimes, ginger pills (available at health food stores) help with nausea induced by anti-Parkinson drugs.

Medications for Constipation

Constipation is a frequent problem among persons with Parkinson disease. There are a large number of over-the-counter remedies for constipation, many of them based on naturally occurring laxatives such as senna leaves or prune juice. Along with a balanced diet, good hydration, and exercise, these natural substances can help with bowel regularity. Over-the-counter stool softeners such as docusate salts can help one maintain a softer stool consistency, which also helps regularity. It is advisable to use mild stool softeners on a regular basis to avoid more severe constipation or even stool impaction. More aggressive laxatives (such as milk of magnesia, glycerin, or enemas) can be habit forming and should only be used if there has been no bowel movement for three to four days. One laxative that seems to work well for people with Parkinson disease when taken on a regular basis is polyethylene glycol (brand name Miralax). If going for many days without a bowel movement is a frequent occurrence despite a regular "bowel program" as described here, the physician should be consulted. As a rule, fiber-containing, bulk-forming laxatives are not encouraged for people living with Parkinson disease. These remedies work only if the person takes sufficient amount of fluids (eight to 10 tall glasses a day). Indeed, not drinking enough fluids while taking these laxatives may have the opposite result, that is, worsening of the constipation.

Antidepressant and Antianxiety Medications

As mentioned in Chapter 4, persons living with Parkinson disease often have to cope with depression and anxiety. Therefore it is not at all unusual for them to be prescribed antidepressant and anxiolytic (antianxiety) medications. In general terms, antidepressants belong in one of two major categories, depending on their chemical structure and mode of action. One category that is very popular with health care providers is the SSRI medications (short for "selective serotonin reuptake inhibitors"). Most people are familiar with the first medication of this class that was ever produced, fluoxetine, better known under the brand name Prozac. These medications act by modifying the processing in the brain of a chemical called **serotonin**, which shares some chemical characteristics with dopamine but is involved more in the experience of emotions and pain rather than in mobility. The second big category is the tricyclic antidepressants, named for their peculiar molecular structure. One widely used medication from this category is amitriptyline (brand name Elavil). These antidepressants are older than the SSRIs and work through another brain chemical, **norepinephrine**. Several studies have shown that these older antidepressants are very effective in treating depression in Parkinson disease—at least as effective as their newer counterparts. In addition to these two categories, other antidepressants are also available, but all of them work through modifying serotonin, norepinephrine, or both.

One common property of all antidepressants is important to keep in mind: their action is not immediate, and the full antidepressant effect may not materialize for several weeks. A number of studies have found that during this early part of the treatment, there may be a slight increase in the risk of suicidal thoughts (or even attempts in some patients), and therefore people who start treatment with antidepressants should be closely monitored for any such feelings. All antidepressants have a variety of side effects. Some tend to cause drowsiness, in which case they may double as mild sedatives in persons who also have insomnia, while others may give people a slight nervousness, similar to a slight "caffeine buzz." The older antidepressants tend to have more nuisance side effects, such as dry mouth, blurred vision, increased constipation, or increased trouble with urination; in serious cases, they can cause urine retention, a dangerous situation. In older persons, especially those who may experience significant cognitive problems, these medications can cause confusion or even hallucinations. There is a concern that because of their mechanism of action, SSRI antidepressants may interact with MAO-B inhibitors such as rasagiline and selegiline to cause a dangerous rise in blood pressure. Therefore such combinations should be used with caution.

Most antianxiety drugs have an addictive potential, an important fact to remember. Just like antidepressants, some anxiolytics may have a sedative effect, but regular use of these medications to induce sleep is not recommended, because they tend to lose their effectiveness with continuous use; that leads to higher doses and eventual dependence on the drug. The most common use of anxiolytics is on an as-needed basis, with strict limits that are not to be exceeded without a careful discussion with the physician. The most widely known drug in this category is diazepam (brand name Valium), although newer, less-sedating anxiolytics, such as alprazolam or lorazepam, are now used. One medication in this category, clonazepam (brand name Klonopin), has a special use in treating the REM sleep behavioral disorder that was mentioned in Chapter 4 and earlier in this chapter. As with most other medications that affect brain chemistry, these drugs can cause confusion, especially in elderly or cognitively affected individuals. They should never be mixed with alcohol, for any reason.

Drugs are not always the best solution to emotional problems such as depression and anxiety. Because of the different ways insurance companies cover mental health problems, often it is the the family physician or the neurologist who decides how to treat such issues. It's always, however, best to ask the experts, and therefore if medications are not effective in alleviating these problems, a consultation with a psychiatrist or possibly a psychotherapist should be pursued.

Medications for Excessive Salivation and for Thick Secretions

Drugs that decrease the amount of saliva also make saliva and other secretions thicker. Because this can be quite uncomfortable, using medications to control drooling is reserved for really severe cases or for special occasions. Some people with Parkinson disease may use drops or pills that reduce salivation as needed, for example, for social outings, for going to church, or when they visit with friends. There are a few different pills, but the most frequently used are glycopyrrolate (brand name Robinul), and hyoscyamine (brand name Levsin); drops may use atropine. All these medications can cause a number of side effects, such as blurred vision, constipation, nausea, erectile dysfunction, decreased sweating, and even irregular heartbeat; therefore they should be used sparingly. Botulinum toxin injections into the salivary glands have also been effective in decreasing saliva production, but on rare occasions they have the unwanted complication of temporarily worsening swallowing.

Some persons with Parkinson have the opposite problem from excessive saliva. They develop thick secretions and have trouble clearing their throat or are bothered by thick postnasal drip. Over-the-counter preparations such as guaifenesin (brand name Mucinex), adequate hydration, and a space humidifier may be helpful measures in this case.

Medications to Improve Bladder Control and Erectile Function

Persons living with Parkinson disease may experience urgency and frequency of urination and often have to get up a lot at night to go to the bathroom. Although a number of medications are effective in treating these symptoms, these same medications may worsen a person's ability to relax the bladder in order to start the urinary stream. In a man with prostate trouble, this can even cause a serious condition, urinary retention. Therefore it's best to first try to manage the bladder symptoms as much as possible without medications. Some of the nondrug treatments are discussed in Chapter 9.

Most medicines used to control this bladder overactivity work by blocking the effect of acetylcholine. If you have read the information presented so far in this chapter, you will have learned that drugs that block acetylcholine may have a number of unpleasant side effects, such as confusion, blurred vision, increased constipation, and dry mouth. Medications commonly used for bladder control include oxybutynin (brand name Ditropan, tolterodine (Detrol), and propantheline (brand name Pro-Banthine), but there are also a number of newer medications in the same category. Sometimes, if starting the urine stream is difficult, doctors may prescribe tamsulosin (brand name Flomax), which may make urination easier but can often cause a drop in blood pressure. Conversely, some of the medications used to keep blood pressure high may make bladder emptying more difficult. One such medication is midodrine, which was discussed earlier, in the section drugs for orthostatic hypotension.

As mentioned in Chapter 4, persons living with Parkinson disease may experience increased difficulties with their sexual abilities. Many people are reluctant to discuss this problem openly. However, a healthy sex life is an important component of a person's quality of life. Since help may be available, it is important to discuss such problems with your doctor. Medications commonly used to treat erectile dysfunction, such as sildenafil (brand name Viagra), vardenafil (Levitra), and tadalafil (Cialis), can be effective in men with Parkinson disease. Three things, however, are very important to know prior to using these medications. First, your doctor will need to review all your other medications. Some medications used in Parkinson disease—for example, propranolol, a beta-blocker sometimes used to treat tremor—may cause erectile dysfunction, so the solution may be as simple as skipping a dose of that medication when anticipating intercourse (but you should *not* skip doses of any medications without permission from your doctor). Second, any psychological factors should be discussed and treated: depression is a common cause of decreased sexual desire and erectile dysfunction. And third, you should have a detailed discussion with your doctor about the risks of using these medications, and you should make sure your doctor is aware of any heart trouble you may have before prescribing them.

Some anti-Parkinson medications, particularly the dopamine agonists pramipexole or Mirapex, and ropinirole or Requip) more than others, may cause increased sexual desire and even obsessing about sex. This can be a serious side effect, as it may create serious difficulties with intimacy in couples affected by Parkinson's. It is important to recognize and discuss such trouble with your doctor. A decrease in dosage may be all that's necessary to deal with this issue, but when the problem is severe, the medication should be discontinued completely. If that's not possible without a serious decline in motor function, then psychiatric medications (antidepressants, anxiolytics, or even antipsychotics) may need to be used to curb the abnormally increased sexual desire.

Medications for Seborrheic Dermatitis and Blepharitis

Hydrocortisone cream, dandruff shampoo, and ketoconazole (brand name Nizoral), a local medication used to treat fungal infections of the skin, are helpful in treating oiliness and flakiness of the skin of the face, eyebrows, and scalp. When the condition spreads to the eyelids (blepharitis), inflammation can be treated with wet, warm compresses (a simple alternative is a warm, wet teabag). Artificial tears may be needed to prevent the inflammation from becoming an infection and spreading to the eye itself. In more severe cases, a dermatologist or ophthalmologist should be consulted.

> Brain surgery has been a risky and variably effective treatment for Parkinson disease for nearly 80 years; however, scientific and technological advances of the last 30 years have turned brain surgery into a very effective treatment for some patients.

Brain Surgery for Parkinson Disease

A Little History and an Overview

It may come as a surprise to learn that brain surgery has been effective in treating the symptoms of Parkinson disease for more than 70 years. Brain surgery for Parkinson's started in the 1930s after physicians noticed that some people with a Parkinson-related tremor were suddenly tremor free after having small strokes. Neurosurgeons and neurologists thought that if they could induce a small, "controlled" stroke or other similar small lesion in certain parts of the brain, they might be able to improve many of the symptoms that make life difficult for people with Parkinson disease. In those early years, there were no effective medications for Parkinson's, so many people with the disease agreed to the surgery—this despite the fact that the success rate of these early procedures was very low, while the rate of serious complications was very high.

Pallidotomy, thalamotomy, and deep-brain stimulation are various forms of **functional neurosurgery** for Parkinson disease.

The rationale behind this brain surgery was that the symptoms of Parkinson stem from an imbalance in the electrical activity of certain brain structures that are charged with controlling movement. This theory is considered valid even today. We discussed in Chapter 2 how the brain, using dopamine, achieves movement control through a sort of "push–pull" mechanism. In Parkinson disease, the lack of dopamine causes too little of the "pushing" or the "pulling" in some brain structures and too much of it in others. The result is that while some neurons become less active or even die, others end up working too much. By silencing these hyperactive neurons, brain surgery rebalances the system and helps control tremors, bradykinesia, and rigidity. This neurosurgical strategy is called **functional neurosurgery**. Early procedures achieved this result either by removing small parts of the brain cortex (the outside part of the brain hemispheres) or by cutting the connection between the brain and muscles by snipping nerve fibers in the spinal cord or the nerve roots as they come out of the spinal column. In the 1940s, the procedure that seemed to be most effective was snipping a bundle of fibers in the brain that connected two groups of neurons in the **basal ganglia** (the structure deep inside the brain that regulates movement). That procedure is called ansotomy.

At about the same time, in the late 1940s, a new approach to doing brain surgery was developed, called **stereotaxic surgery**. In this approach, a probe is lowered into the brain through a small hole in the skull, thereby minimizing the overall brain trauma of the surgery. The probe uses an electric current (heat or freezing may also be used) to make a small, "controlled" lesion, or hole, in the brain tissue surrounding the probe's tip. Detailed brain maps helped doctors calculate the exact track of the probe needed to reach the intended target. This way, neurosurgeons could induce small lesions in deep-brain structures that could not possibly be reached with open-brain surgery (at least not without a high risk of major brain damage). Two new procedures using the stereotaxic technique became popular in the 1950s, called **pallidotomy** and **thalamotomy**. These names derive from the particular brain structure that was lesioned in each (the **globus pallidus**, or **pallidum**, and the **thalamus**, respectively). Although these procedures were sometimes successful, the equipment was not precise, resulting in some patients' having strokes or bleeding in the brain. Also, the chance of putting a lesion in the wrong place was high. So when levodopa appeared in the 1960s, these surgeries became nearly extinct.

In the late 1980s, doctors realized that levodopa was not quite as effective as it had been hoped in patients with advanced stages of Parkinson disease. During the 30 years between the 1950s and 1980s, technology had made wonderful advances. The development of computers allowed for better imaging of the brain ("imaging" is a term that describes all the various types of brain scans), which in turn permitted the construction of better brain maps. Neurosurgeons could now connect the stereotaxic probe to computerized equipment that could instantly analyze the electrical activity of the neurons close to its tip, thereby providing very accurate information as to whether the probe was indeed at the intended target. And scientists had dramatically expanded their understanding of the relationships among the various parts of the basal ganglia, thereby helping them to pick better targets. Scientists also had figured out a new way to silence the hyperactive neurons—by applying a low-intensity, high-frequency current, rather than by killing them with electricity, heat, or freezing. Therefore if the surgery was not effective, at least the wrong brain part was not permanently damaged. All these factors helped minimize complications and maximize the effectiveness of functional neurosurgery for Parkinson disease. In particular, a procedure called deep-brain stimulation (the details of which we discuss later in this chapter) is now frequently used to treat the symptoms of Parkinson disease and some of the complications of its treatment.

> Transplantation of adrenal, fetal, and stem cells are past and proposed forms of **restorative neurosurgery** for Parkinson disease.

Besides functional neurosurgery, doctors have tried to use brain surgery to "cure" Parkinson's. If the reason people get the disease is a lack of dopamine-producing neurons in the substantia nigra, then why not implant dopamine-producing neurons? Wouldn't that fix the problem once and for all? Organ transplantation works for the liver, heart, and kidneys, so why not for brain cells? Surgery for Parkinson disease with this goal is called **restorative neurosurgery**. Finding a restorative procedure that cures Parkinson disease is one of the holy grails of modern medicine. The biggest challenge is, where do you find dopamine neurons to implant? That is, who is the donor? Unlike other cells of our body, neurons do not multiply. We are born with a certain number of neurons and lose some everyday as we age. Other cells in our body get renewed constantly. Our skin, blood cells, and the cells lining our stomach, mouth, and intestines keep multiplying throughout our life. The reason people can afford to donate a part of their liver is that they can grow back the donated portion. Bone marrow transplants are possible because a very small amount of donated bone marrow cells is sufficient to replenish the entire bone marrow of the person receiving the transplant.

So for transplantation of dopamine-producing cells to be possible, a source had to be found that didn't consist of neurons. In the 1980s, scientists tried using a type of cell from the adrenal glands as donor cells. These cells produce a chemical similar to dopamine, called **adrenaline**, and the hope was that implanting these cells in the brain might provide more raw materials from which the brain could make dopamine. Despite early excitement, a large study conducted in the United States did not show any evidence of a consistent benefit from these adrenal transplants. The surgery was soon abandoned. Then doctors looked for a source of *immature* cells that were destined to become dopamine neurons. This led to transplantation of fetal cells: immature nerve cells obtained from the developing brains of human fetuses that had recently died because of miscarriage or selective abortion. Many ethical questions had to be settled before these studies could proceed. In addition, some of the volunteer Parkinson patients had to agree to undergo brain surgery without actually receiving a transplant. Such "sham operations" are necessary so that one can make comparisons between groups of patients who have undergone the exact same procedures except for the treatment under investigation.

The first study of fetal transplants was published in 2001. As a group, patients who received the transplant did not do better than the patients who had sham operations. However, when scientists separated the patients by age, they found that people younger than 60 who had the transplant did better than those who had the sham procedure. Unfortunately, a few months to years after the surgery, some of the successful cases developed dyskinesias similar to those that occur after long-term treatment with levodopa. Although these patients were taking levodopa, their dyskinesias persisted even after levodopa was discontinued. In recent years, enthusiasm about fetal transplants declined even further. One of the "successful" cases died, and scientists were able to look in this person's brain.

They found an unpleasant surprise: Parkinson disease had affected the transplanted cells as well. Nevertheless, a lot was learned from these studies. For one thing, scientists confirmed that grafted cells can survive, produce dopamine, and develop connections with other neurons. Second, in younger patients, there was measurable improvement.

Thus research is continuing, and now scientists are looking into another source of donor dopamine neurons: stem cells. Stem cells are immature cells that have the potential to develop into all kinds of highly specialized cells (as opposed to just neurons). Over the last decade, scientists have been increasing their understanding of the processes that take place for a stem cell to grow into, say, a dopamine-producing neuron. The concept behind restorative neurosurgery with stem cells is that one could implant these cells into the basal ganglia, then coax them into becoming dopamine-producing neurons and developing all the necessary connections, thereby fixing the problem that's causing the disease. Although this sounds promising, the disappointing results of the previous restorative procedures have made scientists cautious about proceeding with experimentation on people before some fundamental questions are answered through animal experiments. Taking the scientific argument one step further, some researchers are asking what would keep whatever is killing a person's dopamine neurons in the first place from attacking the transplanted cells as well. In fact, the case of the fetal-transplantation patient mentioned earlier suggests such an attack may be likely.

It is not the purpose of this book to enter into a discussion of the ethics of stem cell research, beyond pointing out that the use of tissues derived from human fetuses remains highly controversial from a philosophical point of view and is morally highly objectionable to many people. This fact makes it even more imperative that the science proceeds cautiously and that our understanding of the biological and scientific issues is optimized before we can talk about human experimentation.

> **Deep-brain stimulation** works by resetting the balance of the electrical activity of brain structures involved in the control of voluntary movements.

Deep-Brain Stimulation

The most commonly used brain surgery for Parkinson disease is the deep-brain stimulation (DBS) procedure. In a nutshell, in DBS surgery the surgeon inserts a wire (similar to a pacemaker wire) in a certain brain structure (we will discuss which structure below.) Each side of our brain controls the opposite side of our body. So if the symptoms are really bad on the right and quite mild on the left, then inserting the wire in the left side of the brain may be sufficient. When the wire is inserted only in one side of the brain, this is called a unilateral procedure. Most Parkinson's patients who benefit from this surgery will end up needing a wire on both sides (a bilateral procedure). Some neurosurgeons prefer to do a bilateral procedure within one session rather than stagger it over two separate procedures. The wire is placed in its intended position (the target) through a burr hole in the skull, usually an inch or two to the side of and a little forward of the crown. The wire (or wires, for bilateral procedures) is then connected to a battery pack, which is implanted under the skin of the patient's chest, just as with a heart pacemaker. This unit is called the **neurotransmitter** (not to be confused with the chemical neurotransmitters that send signals between neurons). The stimulation can be turned on or off or be adjusted from the outside with a magnet and a specialized computer.

As mentioned earlier, in Parkinson disease some neurons deep inside the brain, in the basal ganglia, become hyperactive from the loss of dopamine. The external stimulation from the deep-brain stimulator silences or suppresses these neurons and in this way resets the balance of the "push–pull" function of the basal ganglia. Such overactive neurons can be found in a structure very close to the substantia nigra, called the **subthalamic nucleus**, as well in the pallidum and the thalamus. The neurologist and neurosurgeon choose one of these three structures to target for DBS depending on the particular symptoms they hope to alleviate. Most people with Parkinson's who undergo this kind of surgery currently get subthalamic stimulation, although studies have shown that pallidal stimulation may be as effective. Thalamic stimulation is reserved for patients in whom tremor is the overwhelming problem, with not much trouble from other symptoms.

The "Ask the Experts" box discusses further details of deep-brain stimulation surgery for Parkinson disease, along with information on who should be considered a good candidate, what are reasonable expectations for the surgery, how to weigh its pros and cons, and a little about the logistics.

Ask the Expert: Should I Have DBS Surgery? What's Involved?

Sierra Farris, PA-C, MPAS, gives us an overview of DBS: "Medications that treat the motor symptoms of Parkinson disease can be effective for many years. But over time, many patients experience a 'wearing off' effect. Many people also eventually experience dyskinesia or involuntary movements. These changes over time can be disruptive to a person's life."One way to minimize or eliminate the wearing-off effect and dys-kinesia is by a treatment called deep-brain stimulation (DBS). DBS is a surgical treatment option for patients who continue to have medication-responsive symptoms. Although brain surgery may sound scary, DBS has improved the lives of thousands of

(Continued)

(*Continued*)

people living with Parkinson's—but does come with the risks of having surgery.

"Here's how it works: Parkinson disease results from diminishing dopamine in the brain, and DBS compensates for the lack of dopamine by stimulating specific areas of the brain with electrical impulses. These microbursts of energy are focused in the globus pallidus internus or the subthalamic nucleus. These areas of the brain send signals that coordinate and control movements.

"The surgical procedure is separated into two stages. In the first operation, a surgeon inserts a DBS lead wire into the brain target after confirming that the location is satisfactory by testing the patient's response to stimulation while awake. This complex, detailed surgery takes several hours. In the second surgery, a neurotransmitter is implanted under the, skin typically in the upper chest area. The neurotransmitter is connected to an extension wire, which is connected to the lead wire. The neurotransmitter is similar in size to a cardiac pacemaker, and like a pacemaker, the neurotransmitter has the purpose of providing constant electrical stimulation to its target. In the case of DBS, the stimulation mimics the effects of medication once the neurostimulator is set to optimal or therapeutic settings.

"After the surgeries are complete and the neurotransmitter is operating at optimal settings—this must be achieved gradually over a period of weeks or months—most patients experience several benefits. One benefit is a significant reduction or complete elimination of the wearing-off effect. Patients using DBS therapy experience much more 'on' time. Another benefit is significant reduction in involuntary movements. And the third benefit, much desired by most patients, is a decrease in the amount

(*Continued*)

(Continued)

of medication needed—many patients end up taking smaller and less frequent doses of drugs.

"A 2006 European study of 156 patients with severe motor complications of Parkinson disease found that 'patients in the DBS group experienced a 25 percent average improvement in quality of life scores, and a 41 percent average improvement in motor function' compared with 'no change on either measure among those patients in the non-DBS group.' The study was published in the New England Journal of Medicine.

"It's important to note that DBS does not cure Parkinson disease. In addition, DBS is not a good treatment for gait freezing, falls, or speech problems. Symptoms that do not respond well to medication won't be helped by DBS. The surgery does not come without risks, including bleeding in the brain, infection, and, infrequently, misplaced wires requiring additional surgery.

"Patients who might be good candidates for DBS are people that can answer 'true' to the following statements:

- 'Levodopa still helps control the movement symptoms of Parkinson disease.' 'My medicine doesn't last from dose to dose or wears off before the next dose is due.'
- 'My medicine still works but isn't controlling my tremor.'
- 'Dyskinesia is limiting my activities, is bothersome, or is causing pain.'
- 'My mind is still sharp, and I am not having hallucinations.'
- 'My mood is not depressed or anxious.'
- 'I don't mind living with an implanted device in my brain or body.' 'My family is supportive, and I can travel for DBS appointments as necessary.'

"After the DBS surgeries, there are few restrictions other than realizing that the DBS device is composed of wires that can

(Continued)

(Continued)

be broken as a result of an accident. Patients must also avoid arc-welding equipment and strong electromagnetic fields. Some medical procedures are not permitted for DBS patients, including body MRIs and therapeutic ultrasound such as diathermy, because of danger of stroke, coma, or death.

"People with joint problems or who may be in need of an MRI should talk to their doctor about getting the MRI prior to DBS surgery. Some MRIs may be performed in people who have had DBS, but only with specialized equipment that's not widely available. Medtronic—the company that manufactures current DBS devices— has customer and technical patient services to answer questions that your health care providers may have about safety issues related to radiology, testing procedures, and surgery in people with DBS.

"Here are questions to ask your neurologist about DBS:
- *'What do you think will improve for me after surgery?'*
- *'Who will program or determine the stimulation settings for me?' (Programming the DBS neurotransmitter requires a skilled, licensed medical professional.)*
- *'How many other patients are you seeing who have one of these devices, and how have they improved with DBS?'*

"Here are several questions to ask a surgeon about DBS:
- *'Is DBS the focus of your practice?'*
- *'How many people have you implanted?'*
- *'Who should I call if I have a problem after I leave the hospital?'*
- *'What is your experience with complications from the surgery?'"*

The Future of Surgery for Parkinson Disease

Deep-brain stimulation is not the last word on surgery for Parkinson disease. In fact, in this chapter we touched only on the "hot issues" on Parkinson surgery. But medicine usually evolves in many different directions simultaneously, and there is no telling which path will lead to the next major breakthrough. Although DBS has been very helpful for a group of people with certain complications of the disease, scientists are still working on finding better targets in the brain where DBS may be beneficial for symptoms not improved by the are currently available procedures. Scientists also are trying to find other ways of using brain surgery to cure the disease. It is beyond the scope of this book to discuss the avenues of research that look promising today, because this information changes rapidly—even as the ink on these pages is drying. New techniques may make use of genetically modified cells or viruses to restore brain chemistry and rebalance neuronal activity. For now, it is enough to remember that every small step counts and that despite not having reached the goal of curing Parkinson disease, the surgical approach to treating it has been a source of otherwise unobtainable knowledge that has dramatically improved our understanding of the disease. Surgery is expected to continue to be a powerful research and treatment tool.

Chapter 8

Disease Management: Rehabilitation Therapy, Assistive Devices, and Adaptive Equipment

In this chapter, we focus on the important role of the rehabilitation team in providing help and assistance for patients and caregivers. Although medications play a primary role in helping to manage the symptoms of Parkinson disease, there is increasing evidence that rehabilitation therapies are also beneficial. As care needs change, many Parkinson's patients seek guidance from physical, occupational, or speech therapists at various times in their journey with Parkinson's. These rehabilitation specialists are trained to improve or maintain functional movement, communication, and involvement in daily life, helping each person to reach her fullest potential.

This chapter will also offer advice on devices and equipment that can make life easier for people with Parkinson disease.

Physical Therapy

Scientific research shows that physical therapy helps Parkinson's patients when added to a standard regimen of medication. Physical therapists are trained professionals who work to improve or restore mobility in their patients while providing ongoing education to ensure patients' understanding and follow-through. Recent laboratory studies have shown that physical exercise may benefit brain function by helping remaining dopamine work more efficiently. These studies also seem to suggest that early addition of physical exercise to Parkinson's treatment provides the greatest benefit. Thus it is important to seek physical therapy evaluation and treatment even in early stages of Parkinson disease to ensure that an appropriate exercise program is added to your daily routine.

> **Physical therapists** work on improving mobility, strength, and balance.

Parkinson disease causes changes in both mobility and perception. People with Parkinson's tend to make slower and smaller motions than people without the disease when walking, bending, or reaching. This smallness of movement, referred to as **hypokinesia**, affects most functional movements and can contribute to shuffling gait, loss of arm swing, and feelings of fatigue. As the motions become smaller, perception is also affected, so that people with Parkinson's begin to feel that these smaller motions are of normal size. Focused attention and practicing larger, exaggerated motions can be helpful in "recalibrating" the brain to achieve full, normal-size movements. People with Parkinson's often benefit from deliberately making their motions "too big" in order to compensate for hypokinesia. Working with a physical therapist on exercises, walking, and functional activities focused on increasing movement size has proven beneficial for many patients.

> Deliberately making **"big" movements** is one technique that helps reduce the hypokinesia caused by Parkinson's.

The series of motions required to rise from a chair or get in and out of bed are learned sequences that we tend to do without conscious thought. Parkinson disease, however, causes difficulty in activating sequences of movement we usually place "on automatic." When the sequence is difficult to activate, these once-simple tasks become increasingly difficult. Physical therapists can help patients perform such tasks by breaking down the sequence and working on each step in the process until it becomes easier.

Parkinson-related muscle stiffness and rigidity has potential long-term complications, including loss of flexibility, reduction in muscle strength, changes in posture, and pain. Physical therapists can recommend stretching exercises and techniques for postural alignment and pain control. Relaxation training may also be used to help reduce stress and muscle tension.

Many patients begin to notice balance changes after living with Parkinson disease for some time. Balance changes may vary with each individual and can present as "freezing," backward loss of balance (also called retropulsion), difficulty turning corners, or falling. A physical therapist can assess balance difficulties and offer instruction on appropriate exercises, balance safety strategies, assistive walking devices to improve safety and reduce fall risk, or some combiniation of theses approaches. If a patient is injured in a fall, physical therapists can work in hospital, transitional-care, home-care, and outpatient settings to help the individual return to his or her preinjury level of function.

Occupational Therapy

An **occupational therapist** helps patients improve the efficiency and safety of their activities of daily living.

Although the word "occupational" might make one think that an occupational therapist helps with on-the-job skills, this skilled professional actually does much more. In truth, occupational therapists help patients better perform numerous kinds of daily tasks. Each person's daily routine is unique, but it usually includes self-care activities like dressing, bathing, brushing one's teeth, and combing one's hair. Many people are involved in household chores that may include cooking, laundry, housekeeping, and yard work. We also tend to drive cars, maintain our finances, manage medication schedules, and do other tasks requiring concentration, memory, handwriting, or typing. Daily life can involve a regular work schedule but also usually involves some pursuit of leisure interests and hobbies. Occupational therapists play a role in helping those with Parkinson's perform all these activities.

A thorough assessment by an occupational therapist will usually include a comprehensive evaluation of arm and hand function, including flexibility, strength, and coordination. The therapist may recommend exercises to improve or maintain function of the upper extremities or may recommend adaptive equipment that allows the person with Parkinson disease to perform a daily task with greater ease.

Task analysis of activities performed in the daily routine will often result in recommendations to improve the ease and safety of such regular activities. For example, an occupational therapist may assess the risk of falling and provide recommendations to reduce this risk as a person moves around the kitchen to prepare a meal or may offer suggestions for installation of bathroom safety equipment to ensure safe bathing and toileting. Some occupational therapists are involved in evaluating work sites to suggest ways to enhance and improve performance of job tasks, while others offer in-depth assessments of safety and vehicle operation while a person is driving.

> Occupational therapists may help **educate care partners** on how to safely provide hands-on assistance to their affected loved ones.

Occupational therapists also offer assessment of and insight into visual, perceptual, or cognitive changes caused by Parkinson disease. If deficits are identified, occupational therapists work with a patient and the patient's family to offer recommendations to lessen or compensate for these deficits. Examples include suggestions to make reading easier or developing a system to keep medications on schedule. An occupational therapy referral may also be helpful for obtaining recommendations for modifying performance of leisure activities and hobbies or to offer suggestions for new areas of interest.

If Parkinson disease results in a significant loss of mobility, occupational therapists are often involved in the assessment and fitting of appropriate wheelchair and seating systems to ensure good positioning, comfort, and to prevent skin breakdown. Education of family members and care partners also becomes important if the person with Parkinson's requires more hands-on assistance to perform daily self-care tasks.

Speech Therapy

An estimated 98 percent of people with Parkinson disease experience changes in communication. Speech pathologists are professionals who specialize in the treatment of speech and language disorders. Research shows that speech therapy treatment can reduce communication deficits caused by Parkinson disease.

A **speech pathologist** can assess and help improve voice strength, slurred speech, swallowing trouble, saliva control, communication, and cognitive functioning.

Changes to the motor and sensory processing systems can affect communication. Many people with Parkinson disease are frustrated by frequent requests to repeat themselves during conversation. One reason is that patients often develop a condition referred to as hypokinetic dysarthria, in which the slowed, smaller motions of people with Parkinson disease affect muscles in the face, lips, and tongue used to produce speech. There can also be smallness of movement in the respiratory system, which provides breath support to produce voice volume. These movement changes result in soft, slurred speech that is often difficult to understand.

Changes in sensory processing can cause people with Parkinson disease to feel they are speaking in a normal audible voice when in fact their speech is soft and difficult to hear. Such individuals often need to exert an effort that feels like shouting to achieve a normal speaking voice. Speech therapy techniques can help them to "recalibrate" their voices so as to turn up the volume and speak appropriately loudly on a consistent basis. Specially trained speech pathologists use a technique called **Lee Silverman Voice Treatment** (or **LSVT**) LOUD, which is based on clinical research, to maximize voice volume in individuals with Parkinson disease.

Speech pathologists also provide comprehensive evaluation and treatment for people experiencing dysphagia, or difficulty swallowing. The speech pathologist will assess swallowing through evaluation of musculature and a review of the person's posture and positioning when eating. Special tests such as a **video swallowing assessment** (a kind of X-ray of the swallowing mechanism) may also be recommended. Treatment may include exercises to improve the swallowing mechanism, recommendations for improved posture and positioning at mealtime, and suggestions for diet modification. The speech pathologist will also discuss and address excessive salivation and techniques to minimize drooling.

For people experiencing changes in memory, concentration, or thought processes, a speech pathologist may become involved in overall assessment and treatment to improve or provide compensation strategies for these cognitive deficits. As Parkinson disease progresses, communication may become more difficult and also more important, because the Parkinson's patients have to be able to communicate about their needs or discomfort. Communication may develop into a source of frustration for both patients and care partners. At this stage, referrals to speech therapy often focus on designing alternative forms of communication or on the use of specialized communication assistive devices.

Assistive Devices and Adaptive Equipment

A variety of useful tools and equipment can make living with Parkinson disease easier. Seeking out this equipment can be somewhat daunting, because there are a myriad of stores, catalogs, and web sites where literally thousands of pieces of equipment are available. It is often helpful to speak with members of your health care team prior to making an equipment purchase, as they have more experience and will be able to provide you with recommendations to ensure that you obtain items that will be useful at the lowest possible expense.

Some equipment (such as walking devices like canes and walkers) may be covered by medical insurance. But choose wisely: a hasty purchase may prove to be a costly mistake.,Many insurance plans will only cover one such device every five years. So before purchasing such equipment, make sure you have reviewed the options carefully and have obtained recommendations from your team, who can offer suggestions and instruction in proper use. Other types of equipment (including adapted silverware, shower benches, and kitchen utensils) are usually *not* covered by insurance. It is easy to order the wrong item because there are many varieties. Make sure your purchase is designed to do what you are hoping, and seek recommendations from your team or from others with Parkinson disease who have experience using that specific item.

Below, we provide answers to many commonly asked questions related to equipment that will make living with Parkinson disease easier.

Where Should Grab Bars Be Installed?

The most important equipment is items that make living in your home safer. Most people living with Parkinson disease would benefit from the installation of safety grab bars in their bathroom near the shower, tub, and toilet. Make sure that these items are installed correctly and securely into the studs of the wall. When moving around the bathroom, avoid using grab bar "substitutes" like soap dishes, faucet handles, and shower rods. These items will easily come off the wall if too much pressure is applied to them, and you could be injured.

In addition to these bathroom modifications, some people have found it beneficial to install a vertical grab bar next to the door of their home either on the inside or on the outside (whichever side the door pulls open from). This provides a sturdy hold and can reduce the risk of backward loss of balance when pulling the door open.

What About Stair Railings?

Stair railings should be installed in all indoor and outdoor stairways in the home. When possible railings should be installed on both sides of the stairs. Make sure railings extend the entire length of the staircase. If the original railing was too short, you may need to add an additional length of railing. In some homes, it may be possible to extend the railing up onto the wall at the top of the stairs. This helps prevent the individual with Parkinson's from bending or stooping excessively to reach down to the rail when descending from the top.

If the person needs support when walking, railings can also be installed in hallways or the bedroom. An accessible ramp may work best for steps into the garage or outdoors.

What Other Types of Equipment Help Promote Bathroom Safety?

Standing in the shower or climbing into a bathtub may prove difficult or unsafe for those with balance changes related to Parkinson disease. Consider purchasing a sturdy shower or tub bench. These items come in several styles. Obtaining a bench with a backrest is often recommended, because it reduces the risk of backward balance loss. Some styles of benches bridge over the side of the tub, allowing the user to first sit down on the outside of the tub before sliding her or his legs across for bathing.

If balance changes require you to take a seated shower, consider buying a simple handheld showerhead, which is easy for most people to use and spray where they want. If you feel safe enough to take a shower standing, be sure to use nonskid strips or a mat in the bottom of the tub.

If rising from a seated position is proving more difficult, an elevated toilet seat may make doing so easier and safer. You can have a higher toilet installed if you are considering renovations or can purchase an elevated seat that can be clamped onto the existing toilet. Avoid molded plastic seats that do not clamp firmly to the sides of the toilet. Some elevated seats have attached armrests for added support, while others require installing a grab bar on the adjoining wall.

You can use a small bench or chair with a backrest next to the bathroom sink when shaving, brushing your teeth, applying makeup, or doing other tasks normally done from a standing position. People who experience frequent backward balance loss will definitely benefit from this adaptation.

Are There Any Other Tips for Bathroom Safety?

- Using "soap on a rope" or installing a body-wash dispenser on the wall prevents having to bend forward to search for dropped soap in the bottom of the tub.
- Some people with Parkinson's find it difficult to dry off after bathing, as muscle rigidity may make it difficult to reach one's back. Don a fluffy terrycloth robe to help absorb moisture and dry off quickly.
- Taped lines in the doorway threshold or a taped "X" in front of the sink or toilet serves as a visual cue to aid people who have freezing episodes in a small, enclosed bathroom space.
- Make sure there is adequate lighting for nighttime trips to the bathroom. Darkened or shadowy rooms promote balance loss and freezing.

How Can I Stay Safer in the Kitchen?

Moving between the counter, stove, sink, table, and refrigerator while preparing food requires frequent stops, starts, and turns. Be mindful of trying to turn corners in a wide arc when moving away from the counter or sink. Place one hand on the counter or shelf when reaching overhead to get items from the cupboard. Consider rearranging your kitchen to place the most commonly used items on the lowest shelf or on the counter. Avoid using step stools to reach into high cabinets.

A number of adaptive cutting boards and knives are available to make food preparation easier. Always make sure you are using good pot holders or oven mitts when cooking on the stove or reaching into the oven. Consider obtaining a kitchen stool or chair to sit on while cooking; this may help you maintain balance. If reaching into the oven becomes too difficult, use a microwave or toaster oven.

Consider buying covered cups and nonglass dishes instead of glass dishes. Practice sliding dishes along the counter or use a small kitchen cart to avoid carrying a lot of things in your hands. (Remember that multitasking becomes difficult with Parkinson disease and sometimes leads to balance loss or falls.)

Work with the occupational therapist on your team to solve specific difficulties you encounter in your own kitchen.

I Am Having Difficulty Rising from a Chair. Would a "Lift Chair" Work for Me?

Chairs with an electric-lift component slowly raise a person from a seated to a near-standing position. In many cases, this is an appropriate option to ensure safety and independence. While some people are concerned that they may become "dependent" on the chair, it does not have to be used consistently. However, it can be very useful when one needs to get up more quickly (as when answering the door or the telephone). An electric-lift chair may also be good for people experiencing motor fluctuations that result in difficulty rising at some times but not others.

Medical equipment companies and some furniture stores carry electric-lift reclining chairs. They come in a variety of shapes and sizes. If possible, go to the store and try sitting in the chair to assess its comfort and how it suits your posture prior to purchase.

Some medical insurance plans provide a stipend for purchasing electric-lift chairs if one has a letter of medical necessity. Check with your plan to find out if this is an option for you and what information needs to be submitted prior to purchase. If your insurance does not help pay for the chair and finances are an issue, consider buying a used chair advertised in the classified section of a newspaper or online.

Is There Equipment to Make Mobility at Night or in Bed Easier?

Many people with Parkinson's have difficulty turning in bed at night because muscle rigidity and slowness affect their legs, arms, and trunk. The reduction in medication over the nighttime hours may also make moving in bed more difficult. Simple strategies like using a satin-based fabric through the middle third of the bed or wearing silk or acetate fabric nightwear make rolling easier. Full satin sheets, however, are often too slippery, offering poor foot traction on the bed.

For some people, a half-side rail or bed pole provides a sturdy grip and makes getting in and out of bed easier. Make sure any device you use is attached firmly and will support your weight during the position change. Avoid half-side rails that are too long, preventing you from easily getting your hips in and out of bed. Overhead bed trapezes often do not work well, because they do not allow you sufficient leverage to get your legs moving.

Good lighting is essential when getting up at night. Shadows or darkened rooms create the potential for balance loss and falls. Consider having an easily accessible lamp or a motion-detector night-light if you do not like to have lights on while sleeping

Some people experience the frequent need or urge to urinate at night, resulting in multiple hurried trips to the bathroom. Consider buying a bedside urinal or commode to make this need easier to accommodate.

Do I Need a Hospital Bed?

Hospital beds are usually used only by people with significant mobility problems who need especial assistance with transfers and bed mobility. These beds usually come with side rails. Some beds are electric and have a remote control to adjust the bed height or to raise the head or foot of the bed (or both). Other beds have a manual crank mechanism to make these adjustments. Check with your insurance plan to see what type of bed it may cover. (Figure 8–1 shows a hospital bed with some useful features.)

Foam mattress pads or electric alternating-pressure pads for hospital beds can be obtained for people with severe mobility problems and the potential for skin breakdown.

Retail stores and online sellers also offer a number of beds that are not hospital beds but have mechanisms for adjusting the bed into a number of positions.

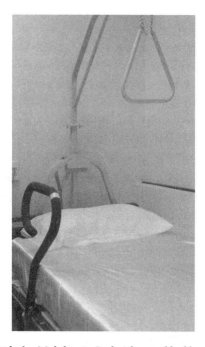

FIGURE 8-1 Aids for Mobility in Bed. *A hospital bed has controls for raising the back or the legs. Parkinson's patients find the type of rail attachment shown at lower left easier to use than the standard bedrails that come with a hospital bed. The bright tape provides a visual cue that may be especially important if a person's vision is affected. Bedclothes of satin or similar slippery fabric improve mobility in bed. This bed has a trapeze overhead, which is not very helpful to people with Parkinson's.*

Is There Equipment to Make Getting in and out of the Car Easier?

Satin-based fabric or a cushion may make it easier to slide into and out of a car. A small tool called a Handybar can also help; it fits into a slot on most cars to creates a handrest one can use when rising. Some people have used a suction-grip grab bar on the top of the car as an added way to stabilize themselves during the transfer.

If you're considering purchasing a new car, don't buy one with low seats that make rising more difficult. Choose leather or vinyl over cloth seats, which often make it more difficult to scoot over. Built-in lumbar support in the seats may also help with posture and positioning when riding.

If you use a wheelchair at all times, you can get a van fitted with an electric lift that allows you to be transported in the chair.

A physical therapist or occupational therapist can work with you to make car transfers safer and easier.

What Do I Do If Car Transfers Do Not Seem Safe or Feasible for My Care Partner to Perform with Me?

Investigate special transportation services in your community. Most of these services will provide transport to medical appointments and other events with advance notice and scheduling. Fees vary based on the vendor and services available in your community.

Are There Practical Ways to Reduce the Risk of Injury from Falling?

If you are falling frequently in your home environment, it may be helpful to look at your home with a fresh eye and remove items that may cause injury in a fall. Obtaining knee and elbow pads for joint protection may also prove beneficial. Other practical suggestions for home safety include the following:

- Remove throw rugs, the most common "fall hazard."
- Get rid of "floor clutter" that may contribute to tripping. Plant stands, footstools, magazine racks, and other low objects can all be hazardous.
- Rearrange furniture to create wide walking paths. Removing the coffee table from the center of the room can open up the space and reduce the risk of falls.
- Reduce the temptation to "climb" by removing footstools and ladders.
- Install vertical grab bars next to doors that pull toward you to minimize the risk of backward balance loss.
- Add lighting to ensure safe nighttime trips to the bathroom.
- Wear shoes with good support, low heels, and nonslip soles.
- Make sure your tub or shower has a nonslip mat.
- Avoid stepping over sleeping pets. Make sure your dog or cat is not underfoot before beginning to move.

How Much Should I Invest in Modifying My Home?

Home renovation or modifications can be time-consuming and expensive. Before undertaking a major remodeling project, ask yourself a few questions: How long do I plan to stay in my current home? Will the modifications I make allow me to continue to live here? Do I have the financial resources to complete the renovation project?

If you decide to start the remodeling project (or if you are moving to a new space and have choices in the finishing process), there are several options to consider:

- Low-pile carpeting without excessive patterns or wood or laminate flooring is usually best for safe walking if you plan to use an assistive device or wheelchair.

- Make doorways wider if you use an assistive device or wheelchair or may need to do so in the future.
- Walk-in showers allow one to bathe without having to step over the edge of a tub.
- Shower curtains often are easier to move around than solid shower doors.
- Elevated toilets make transfer easier.
- Wide walking paths throughout the residence, without tight corners or excessive furniture, make mobility easier.
- Ramps may be installed in place of stairways, or electric "stair glides" may be installed to enable one to negotiate stairs safely.
- When possible, create "one-level living"; that is, have the bedroom, bathroom, and living space all on one floor.
- A ramp or one-level living can make it easier to access the outdoors.
- Have a place where a care partner or live-in assistant can sleep within easy access or hearing distance of the person with Parkinson's if needed.

What Assistive Device Can Make My Walking Safer?

There are a variety of gait assistive devices designed to promote safe walking and minimize loss of balance. It is highly recommended that you seek input from a physical therapist before purchasing such a device. Doing so will help ensure that you receive the most appropriate device, that it is adjusted to an appropriate height, and that you have received instructions in its proper use.

What Assistive Devices Do *Not* Typically Work Well for People with Parkinson Disease?

Generally, any assistive device that interrupts the normal flow of walking may hinder someone with Parkinson disease. Since people with Parkinson's typically walk with short, shuffling steps and have difficulty starting and stopping, devices like standard four-post walkers and quad canes (canes with a four-legged base) do not work well. Many people with Parkinson's who attempt to use these devices tend to "carry" them along without setting the legs firmly on the ground. This does not enhance walking stability and may actually promote loss of balance. Although well-meaning friends and family may try to loan you these devices, avoid using them. It's best to ask a physical therapist what device is best for you.

So What Device May Best Aid My Walking?

Someone experiencing mild balance imprecision when walking or feelings of balance loss on uneven terrain may benefit from the use of a single-end cane or walking stick. These assistive devices do not interrupt the normal flow of walking, and their tips can be set down on the ground to widen the base of support, minimizing loss of balance.

Canes should be adjusted to allow 15–30 degrees of bend at the elbow when one is gripping the cane. When walking, the cane should be set firmly on the ground and not carried. A patient can work with a physical therapist to learn proper technique.

Many people have found that aluminum or wood walking sticks, also known as hiking poles, provide balance support while enabling more upright posture. They are particularly helpful when one is walking on uneven terrain (grass, gravel, uneven sidewalks, etc.). For best stability one can use one or two poles. Hiking poles can usually be found at sporting goods stores. Again, seek instruction from a physical therapist for proper fitting and best use.

If a person needs additional walking support, a wheeled walker typically works best. Aluminum walkers with straight wheels on the front often are difficult to turn and may not offer adequate stability for longer distances or when outdoors. Consider adding swivel casters (the 5-inch size typically works best) to make turning safer with these devices. Glide brakes can also be added to allow safer stops.

Most people who require a walker find that one with four large wheels, swivel casters, hand brakes, and a bench seat (as shown on the left side of Figure 8-2) offers the greatest stability. Walkers like this easily move and turn. Make sure to choose a walker with a sturdy frame and good brakes. Tall individuals or those with large frames may require heavier-duty metal walkers designed for such people. The bench seat can double as a tray space to carry items while walking, and most walkers of this style also come with a basket or bag for other items. If you fatigue easily or have dizziness or fainting spells, the attached seat may be extremely useful, allowing you to sit down when needed.

There is a specialty walker designed specifically for those with movement disorders like Parkinson disease. The U-Step Walking Stabilizer (shown on the right side of Figure 8-2) has a heavy, very

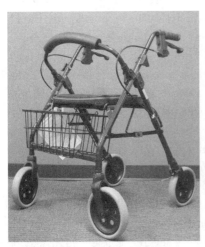
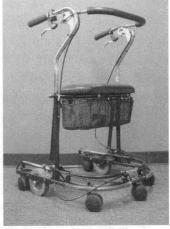

FIGURE 8-2 Gait Assistive Devices. Left: Four-wheel walker with hand brakes, carrying basket, and bench seat. Right: U-Step Walking Stabilizer™.

sturdy frame with multiple casters on a U-shaped base. It also has a "reverse brake" mechanism, meaning that it stays in a locked position until the user releases it by squeezing the hand brake. Tension can be added to the walker to reducing the speed of the device, which may be most helpful to individuals who experience bursts of speed when walking.

It is important to consider the portability of any assistive device. Some walkers are significantly heavier than others and may be difficult to lift into the trunk or backseat of a car. It is advisable to practice folding and lifting any assistive device prior to purchase to ensure that the person with Parkinson's or a family caregiver can safely lift and handle the device for transport.

Consult a physical therapist familiar with all these gait assistive devices to help you select the right one and ensure that it is adjusted and used properly.

When Should I Consider Using a Wheelchair?

Wheelchairs are rarely needed in the early and moderate stages of Parkinson disease. Use of a wheelchair is usually considered if mobility problems are preventing an individual from fully participating in home or community activities. While making the decision to use a wheelchair is often difficult, it is important to recognize that limiting one's activities is isolating, has a negative impact on quality of life, and may actually compromise independence and safety.

Some people choose to use a wheelchair only for going longer distances, attending social events, or shopping. In these cases, the wheelchair can help in combating fatigue and can allow the person to become more fully engaged in the activity. Obtaining a lightweight transport chair that can be easily lifted into and out of the trunk of a car may work best for these situations.

If balance and mobility are more severely challenged, it may be necessary to obtain a wheelchair for more consistent use. When choosing a wheelchair it is important to work with a rehabilitation therapist or vendor with expertise in the options available and trained in appropriate fitting. Options like reclining chair backs, removable leg and arm rests, brake extenders, seating cushions, and trunk supports should all be considered prior to a wheelchair purchase. Make sure the vendor provides information about and support for repair and maintenance of the chair.

The care partner should also have input to ensure the chair will fit within the home environment and can be disassembled and lifted safely into and out of the trunk of a car or van.

Can I Use an Electric Wheelchair or Scooter?

Many people think that the use of an electric device will solve their mobility problems. All too often, they are disappointed after a hastily made purchase. Electric wheelchairs and scooters are very heavy and may not be able to be broken down for transport, so that one has to purchase a van with an electric lift to go from place to place. These devices are also quite large and may not be able to be maneuvered safely at home. Some senior apartment complexes prohibit use of electric scooters and wheelchairs because of potential safety risks to others.

It is important to recognize that Parkinson disease causes not only physical but also cognitive and perceptual challenges that may prevent an individual from operating an electric device safely. Motor fluctuations, excessive dyskinesia, freezing, postural instability, and changes in thinking and memory can all contribute to unsafe operation of motorized devices.

We strongly recommend that a person's abilities be evaluated by a physical or occupational therapist before the purchase of a wheelchair or scooter.

What Adaptations Can Make Eating Easier?

Changes in fine motor coordination and tremor can cause difficulties in cutting food, bringing food from the plate to your mouth, or drinking from a cup. These difficulties can cause frustration and keep people from enjoying social outings at restaurants with friends and family. Some of these frustrations can be reduced by asking for a steak knife to make cutting easier or asking for meat to be cut in the kitchen prior to serving.

There are also a number of adapted eating utensils that can make mealtime easier (see Figure 8–3). "Rocker knives" allow you to cut food in a rocking motion, improving ease and reducing stress. Large-handled utensils may also make eating easier. Curve-handled forks and spoons make it easier to bring food to the mouth without spilling. Plate guards create a ledge on the plate for people who have difficulty loading food onto a fork or spoon. Before purchasing such utensils, talk to an occupational therapist about what options might work best for a particular situation or condition.

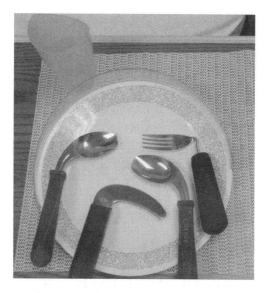

FIGURE 8–3 Adapted Eating Utensils. Clockwise from upper left are a "nosey cup," plate guard, right-handed curved fork and spoon, "rocker knife," and a left-handed curved spoon, all sitting on a nonslip mat.

Covered cups are readily available and can reduce spills related to tremor. If you have difficulty tipping your head back to drink easily, try a "nosey cup," which has a dip in one side so that the nose doesn't block the cup.

Are There Devices That Can Help My Communication?

We live in a high-tech society that has created a number of computerized devices designed to enhance communication. Many of these devices are very expensive and may not offer the consistent performance desired for ongoing use. The individual using the communication device needs to have adequate perception, cognition, and in some cases hand coordination to use it efficiently. Please consult with a speech pathologist familiar with voice-activated and other electronic communication devices before making a purchase.

If an electronic device does not appear to be the answer, the speech pathologist can help you to work with low-tech devices such as word or letter boards, hand signals or gestures, or other strategies for ongoing communication between the patient and the care partner or others. Simple strategies like facing each other when speaking or reducing distracting noise in the environment are often helpful as well.

I Am Having Difficulty Remembering to Take My Pills on a Regular Schedule. What Can Help Me?

It is essential for people with Parkinson's to take their medications on time. Multiple dosing throughout the day can sometimes make it difficult to remember to take pills at the right time. Figure 8–4 shows several devices that are useful for reminding one to take pills.

Putting pills into pill organizers designed for this purpose can help a person stay on track. These boxes can be purchased at most pharmacies. Look for a box that can accommodate the pills in your

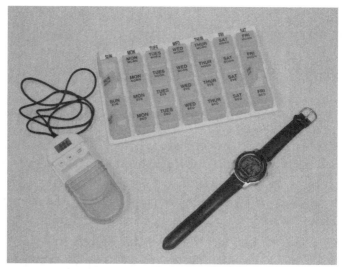

FIGURE 8-4 Devices for Remembering to Take Pills on Time. Clockwise from left are a timer-equipped pillbox, pill organizer, and alarm watch.

regular schedule for a full day. If you are forgetting to take your pills even after setting up a pill organizer, a timer can provide a useful reminder. Some pillboxes have a built-in timer that can be set to regular intervals, creating a beeping or buzzing sound as a reminder that it is "pill time." Some people use an alarm watch that can be set for several times throughout the day. In place of a sound, some watches can create a vibrating sensation on your wrist, alerting you that it is pill time without creating a disturbance in your surroundings.

If you are unsure as to what system will work best for you, a nurse or occupational therapist can review the options and help you make the best choice.

What Adaptations Can Be Made to My Computer?

There are a number of adaptations that can enhance computer use. Computers can be set up to minimize letter repetitions resulting from repeated keystrokes due to slowness or tremor. It is also possible to set up voice-activated typing on your computer. Larger keyboards and monitor screens may also make computer use easier. Check with your occupational therapist about referral sources for adapted-computer services in your area.

Chapter 9

Disease Management: Specific Symptoms

As mentioned in Chapters 3 and 4, people living with Parkinson disease may have to deal with a great variety of symptoms over the years. Naturally, in the earliest stages of the disease, the focus is on the motor problems: tremor, slow movement, and muscle stiffness. Generally, these symptoms respond adequately to medications that replenish the missing dopamine or provide a good substitute for it. As the disease progresses, balance may become more of a challenge, or patients may experience motor complications in the form of dyskinesias or wearing off. Fine-tuning of pill doses and a more complicated medication regimen may provide relief, but it is usually at this stage that patients begin to realize that they have to learn to live with some symptoms and that they may have to "pick their battles" about which symptoms are most important to treat and which to leave alone. It is also at this stage that with the increasing complexity of the drug regimen, more side effects may arise. As the disease spreads in the brain, new symptoms may appear, such as confusion, dementia, hallucinations, and falling.

Most of these challenges in the advanced stages of the disease are not dopamine related, and dopamine drugs not only are useless in dealing with them but may even aggravate them. What's more, for many of these symptoms available medications either are ineffective or may be contraindicated because they can dramatically worsen mobility when given to a person with Parkinson's.

Many of the symptoms in advanced Parkinson disease do not respond to drugs that act on the dopamine system. In fact, such medications may aggravate a lot of these symptoms.

In this chapter we will discuss some of the challenging symptoms of Parkinson disease, from the earliest to the more advanced stages. Because medications have already been discussed in Chapter 7, the focus will be not so much on medications but rather on how can one learn to live with, or manage, some of these challenges. Surprisingly to some, many of the symptoms for which we do not have a "magic pill" respond to therapy intervention. With "compensatory" techniques, one can learn how to overcome a specific challenge by relying on one's strengths or by learning new ways to perform specific tasks. With "restorative" techniques, one can train to strengthen one's weaker areas. It may also come as a surprise to many that such strategies are very important and effective in disease management from the earliest stages. In fact, many specialists in the field of Parkinson disease believe that early involvement with therapy and exercise can result in a strong foundation that will come handy in the later stages of the disease.

Also in this chapter we will discuss how to deal with special circumstances. For example, what should a person with Parkinson disease know about having elective surgery or expect when hospitalized for some other illness in order to anticipate situations that might otherwise create unpleasant surprises?

Managing Tremor, Bradykinesia, and Rigidity

Parkinson's symptoms can fluctuate throughout the day depending on medication levels, fatigue, stress levels, and sometimes unknown reasons. Consider medication schedules when planning your daily routine, opting to do more complex tasks at times when your medication is functioning at its best. Allow adequate time to accomplish tasks and avoid hurrying. Schedule breaks as needed—tasks that you accomplished easily in the past may need to be broken down into several shorter sessions with rest in between. Remember that feelings of stress may make symptoms like tremor and slowness feel even worse. It is usually best to be proactive and plan ahead to reduce feeling hurried or rushed. Start to get ready for scheduled appointments and events well in advance of your departure time.

Small, cramped handwriting (micrographia) can create difficulty and added stress in the daily routine. Figure 9–1 shows several tools that can help with handwriting. It can be helpful to use a large-grip pen and slow down when writing, focusing on making large, exaggerated letters. Printing rather than using a cursive form of writing

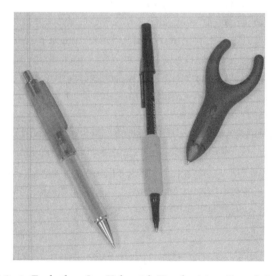

FIGURE 9–1 Tools that Can Help with Handwriting. From left to right are a "fat" pen, a pen with an added grip, and a specialty pen for a modified grip, all sitting on lined paper.

also sometimes helps. Some people find that lined paper helps provide a visual cue for keeping letter sizes larger. To avoid stress when attempting to write a check while standing in a long checkout line with people behind them, some people use a check card or partially fill in check blanks before going to the store. If tremor interferes with writing or other activities that require a steady hand, sometimes wearing a weighted wristband (available in stores selling exercise gear) can help.

Seek out tools and adaptive equipment to make life easier. Button hooks, Velcro closures, elastic shoelaces, long shoehorns, and reachers, can make dressing less cumbersome (Figure 9–2). Jar openers, cutting boards, and other kitchen gadgets reduce frustrations during meal preparation. Large handles on forks, toothbrushes, combs, and other personal items often make them easier to use in the daily

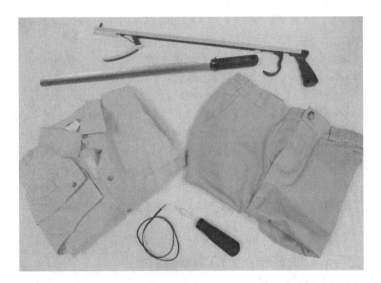

FIGURE 9-2 Clothing and Devices that Make Dressing Easier. At left and right are a shirt and pants with fake buttons and Velcro™ closures; At the bottom there is an elastic shoelace (left) and a buttonhook (right). At the top a reacher and a long-grip shoe horn.

routine (See Chapter 8 for more details on adaptive equipment). Covered cups can help decrease spills caused by tremor. Use of a steak knife or adapted "rocker knives" to make cutting foods easier. Ask for meat to be precut in the kitchen when dining at a restaurant if this is an issue for you. An occupational therapist can help you sort through the array of adaptive equipment on the market and make recommendations on what is most appropriate to your situation.

Be aware that mobility may decline during the nighttime hours, when you are less likely to be taking medication. As discussed in Chapter 8, "slippery fabric" nightwear or satin-based fabric through the middle third of the bed can make rolling easier. Use adequate nighttime lighting for trips to the bathroom. Speak with your medical provider if you experience significant changes in nighttime mobility. Medication adjustments may help remedy this problem. Rehabilitation therapists can also teach safe and effective strategies to make bed mobility easier and can make recommendations for equipment such as a half-side rail or bed pole as needed.

Change position frequently throughout the day to reduce feelings of stiffness and muscle rigidity. Try to do occasional stretches for your neck, shoulders, and trunk if you are sitting in a chair or at a desk or computer for long periods. Use of a lumbar-support cushion in the chair or car can improve sitting posture and reduce back tension and stiffness. The "slippery fabric" concept can also work with getting in and out of a car. Some people find that putting a plastic bag (a trash bag works well) on the car seat reduces friction and makes it easier to swing the legs in and out of the car.

Managing Balance Challenges and Freezing of Gait

Balance changes in Parkinson disease can increase the likelihood of falling. Reduce the risk of falls by creating a safe home environment.

Place frequently used items within easy reach, remove throw rugs, place nonskid bath strips or bathmats in the bottom of the tub, and install grab bars in strategic locations near the toilet and tub or shower. Create safer habits by avoiding climbing on ladders and footstools and by sitting down to dress or shower.

Falls also increase with multitasking. Avoid carrying items in both hands and eliminate distractions when concentrating on tasks that require you to maintain balance while standing and walking.

Some people with Parkinson's experience the frustration of sudden immobility, feeling that their feet are glued to the floor. This phenomenon, known as freezing, can contribute to balance loss and falling. Compensation strategies such as imagining that you are stepping over an imaginary line or kicking through an imaginary wall of glass are often effective means to break out of the freeze. Counting a rhythmic cadence before starting to move may also prove helpful. Marching in place with knees lifted high or rocking from side to side can help "unglue" feet and make stepping or turning easier. It is important to remain calm and avoid hurrying, which can make freezing even worse. See a physical therapist for more comprehensive evaluation of the problem and to create strategies that work best for you.

Injuries and fractures as a result of falling often lead to greater difficulty with mobility and safety. Talk to your physician about receiving a bone density test and obtaining medications for prevention and treatment of osteoporosis (decrease in bone mass and structure that makes bones weaker and more likely to break). To minimize the risk of osteoporosis, eat a balanced diet rich in calcium (found in milk, yogurt, cheese, and calcium-fortified juices and cereals). Vitamin D helps the body absorb calcium, and can be made through exposure to sunlight. If you are housebound or live in a northern, cold-weather climate, a vitamin D supplement may be recommended. Weight-bearing exercises also help bones retain calcium and reduce the risk of osteoporosis.

Dizziness is a symptom that affects balance safety and contributes to falling. Some people use the term "dizziness" to describe feeling unsteady on their feet, while others report feeling as if the whole room is spinning around them. Words like "lightheadedness," "wooziness," or "vertigo" may also be used to describe this symptom. A variety of things may contribute to dizziness, including the following:

- **Low blood pressure:** Parkinson disease and the medications frequently given for treatment of Parkinson's can lower one's standing blood pressure. It is recommended that individuals with Parkinson's routinely have their blood pressure monitored in both sitting and standing positions. (More on this can be found in Chapters 4 and 7 and later in this chapter.)

- **Taking multiple medications:** Taking four or more medications significantly increases the risk of side effects, including dizziness. Make sure your physician is aware of all medications you are taking and be sure to ask questions about potential side effects when starting a new prescription.

- **Inadequate fluid intake:** Dehydration can result in dizziness and loss of balance. Make sure you are drinking enough fluids, particularly during hot, humid weather or if you have been experiencing nausea, vomiting, or diarrhea.

- **Stress and anxiety:** Stress reactions can cause physical symptoms, including feelings of dizziness. Use relaxation techniques like deep breathing, soft music, or guided imagery if you are feeling stressed.

- **Use of alcohol:** Alcoholic beverages affect equilibrium and balance. Limit alcohol intake to reduce the risk of dizziness or falls.

- **Other medical conditions:** Inner-ear disturbances, cardiac problems, diabetes, and depression are just a few of the many other medical conditions that may cause dizziness to occur.

Dizziness may be treated with medications, safety strategies, rehabilitation therapies, and good nutrition. It is important to report feelings of dizziness to your physician, who can make recommendations about the best options to treat your situation.

Managing Weakness and Fatigue

Some people with Parkinson disease report feelings of muscle weakness, even when testing reveals their strength to be quite good. Slowing of motion coupled with muscle rigidity can reduce momentum and effective movement, which contributes to feelings of weakness. Some studies suggest that individuals with Parkinson disease may have reduced core strength in the trunk and abdomen. Reduced activity and an inactive lifestyle can also contribute to loss of strength. Reports of fatigue are almost universal in people with Parkinson disease and can combine with strength losses to further reduce activity levels.

Balancing activity and rest can help reduce fatigue and enhance energy. It can be helpful to set up regular rest periods and avoid "overdoing." Create an activity routine that includes both stretching and strengthening exercises. Focus on large, exaggerated movements while exercising and throughout your daily routine, because small, ineffective motions burn energy and contribute to feelings of fatigue. If tasks like getting out of bed or rising from a chair seem difficult, separate the movement sequence into step-by-step components, focusing on each step as you perform it. A referral to physical or occupational therapy can be helpful to maximize strength and learn strategies for energy conservation.

Decide what is feasible and safe for you to perform, seeking assistance as appropriate. If feelings of weakness coincide with "off periods" related to "wearing off" of the medication, consult your physician for assistance and recommendations.

Managing Dyskinesia, Dystonia, and Wearing Off

Parkinson's medication schedules are complex, and some people notice periods of reduced effectiveness during the day or experience side effects such as dyskinesia and dystonia. It is important to take your medications on a regular schedule as prescribed by your physician. You may wish to keep a log or diary about your symptoms to share with your doctor. This can be an effective way to establish patterns of medication effects and give your physician important information for adjusting your medication schedules.

It is usually best to plan to rest and avoid strenuous activity or exercise during "off times." Use good judgment if dyskinesia affects your balance safety or driving, and avoid unsafe activities. Note that attempts to stop involuntary movements by sitting on a hand, crossing the legs, or other constraints can sometimes contribute to muscle pain and discomfort. Mild stretching can sometimes help alleviate feelings of muscle cramping.

Managing Speech and Communication Problems

Loss of voice volume and imprecise speech articulation can produce communication difficulties. Reducing background noises can help eliminate "competition" and make your voice heard more easily. It may be helpful to sit face to face with the listener when talking. Take deep breaths and practice using your strongest voice when speaking, even if it feels too loud for normal conversation. See a speech pathologist for thorough voice evaluation and treatment.

The expression "you can't judge a book by its cover" can easily be applied to people with Parkinson disease. Reduced facial expression can lead to changes in communication, as most of us rely on facial expressions and gestures to interpret both the speaker's (if we are a listener) and the listener's (if we are the speaker) mood and understanding of what is being communicated. Loss of these automatic responses can be misinterpreted as disinterest, depression, or lack of understanding. Family care partners should be aware that they may need to ask direct questions about how a person with Parkinson's is feeling rather than making assumptions based on facial expressions or body postures.

Just like slowness in movement, people with Parkinson disease can experience slowness in thought processing (**bradyphrenia**). People with Parkinson disease may find it more difficult to respond rapidly to questions or feel that it takes longer to collect their thoughts before speaking. A quiet environment with fewer distractions is sometimes helpful in these situations. The "gift of time" also proves helpful in allowing the person with Parkinson disease to express themselves. Family care partners may need to avoid the tendency to "jump in" and answer for their loved one, as interruptions often make the person's thought process even more difficult.

Managing Excessive Salivation, Drooling, and Thick Secretions

Loss of automatic swallowing causes many people with Parkinson's to feel they have excessive saliva and occasional drooling. Sipping liquids throughout the day will ensure adequate fluid intake and promote active swallowing. Chewing gum or sucking on hard candy can also promote swallowing, but make sure the swallow mechanism works well before using these options. Avoid sugary foods, which cause increased saliva production. Some literature suggests using dried papaya, papaya juice, or even a small amount of meat tenderizer (which consists mainly of dried papaya) swabbed under the tongue to help dry excess secretions. If thick secretions persist, drinking warm broth may help.

Severe drooling can sometimes be helped by medical interventions, including medications or injections (there is more on this in Chapter 7). Consult your physician or a speech pathologist for more information on these and other options to see if they may be appropriate for you.

Managing Swallowing Problems

Approximately 50 percent of people with Parkinson's experience dysphagia (difficulty swallowing). If swallowing problems are mild, they may be helped by making appropriate menu choices, choosing foods that are soft and easy to chew. Avoid foods that are hard to swallow or have crumbly textures. Eat slowly, emphasizing a deliberate swallow or a "double swallow" after each bite. Alternating liquids and solids is sometimes effective. Some people use ice chips or lemon ice between bites to help facilitate swallowing. Try using applesauce or a bit of jelly to help pills slide down more easily. Avoid taking levodopa with substances containing protein, like pudding, yogurt, or ice cream, as these foods may interfere with proper absorption of the medication into your bloodstream.

If swallowing becomes more difficult or you are experiencing frequent coughing or choking, seek referral to a speech pathologist, who can provide more comprehensive evaluation and recommendations for treatment.

In the more advanced stages of Parkinson disease, choking may become quite dangerous, even life-threatening. When foods and fluids slide down "the wrong pipe" they may end up in the lungs and cause an infection, called aspiration pneumonia. In persons in the end stages of the disease, aspiration may happen "silently," that is, without the patient's realizing that it happened, and lead to repeated severe pneumonias. In these cases, the doctor may discuss with the patient and their care partners the option of a **gastrostomy**. This is a surgical procedure that introduces a tube into the stomach through the abdominal wall so that nutrition and hydration can be provided to the individual while bypassing the mouth and esophagus, where aspiration usually happens. Some people may object to such "drastic" measures, and a careful conversation with the doctor is necessary. There is no universal answer as to when and whether such aggressive treatments are appropriate. The person's current quality of life, the discomforts involved or anticipated with or without the procedure, and other aspects of the person's situation have to be examined in detail before a decision can be made.

Managing Vision Problems

Multiple vision problems can occur in Parkinson disease. These include blurred vision, dry eyes, sensitivity to bright light, difficulty reading, and changes in contrast sensitivity (difficulty with vision in low-light conditions). The following are some practical strategies for coping with vision changes:

- Use artificial tears or other lubricating eyedrops regularly.
- Try using a reading magnifier or consider using large-print books or books on tape.
- Individuals with reduced vision may use contrasting colors to more easily see food on their plate, define the edge of stairs, or outline proper hand placement on a grab bar.
- Wear protective eyewear in bright light.
- Always have plenty of light to read by.
- Consult with your eye doctor about what kind of lenses to use in your eyewear. Bifocals, trifocals, and progressive lenses may increase the tendency for double vision and blurred vision in persons with Parkinson disease.

Ask the Experts: Managing Constipation

Susan Imke, GNP-C, says: "Both Parkinson disease and the medications given to treat Parkinson's can aggravate 'gut' problems. Maintaining good bowel function can be challenging, especially
(Continued)

(Continued)

for older adults whose activity levels may be limited. The following are some suggestions:

- *"Increase water consumption to six 8-ounce glasses per day. The role of getting enough water each day in preventing constipation cannot be overemphasized. Seltzer water or club soda adds air as well as moisture to the bowel, which can increase intestinal motility.*
- *"Reduce red meat and dairy products in the diet. Limit high-fat and high-sugar foods; increase fruits and vegetables. A fruit-only snack at night and first thing each morning helps stimulate bowel action.*
- *"Increase exercise and activity levels to help keep things moving!*
- *"Drinking 6 ounces (three-quarters of a cup) of hot tea or hot water with lemon juice on arising each morning can act as a bowel stimulant. Prune juice with pulp can be helpful.*
- *"Stool softeners containing docusate sodium or an Ayurvedic combination called triphala, can be used regularly. Bulking agents such as Metamucil and Citrucel provide a good fiber supplement to the diet but should not be used unless a minimum of 48 ounces of water is consumed throughout the day.*
- *"Stimulant laxatives should ideally be avoided. These products contain stronger agents, with directions to 'take at bedtime to produce a bowel movement in the morning.'*
- *"Some patients report very good results with polyethylene glycol (brand name Miralax), taken as directed. It is now available over the counter, but its use should be approved by your doctor or nurse-practitioner.*
- *"If these measures are not enough to prevent or manage chronic constipation, your physician can recommend prescription medications to use for a limited time.*
- *"Try not to sit on the toilet for longer than five minutes or strain to pass hard stool. The goal is to honor the body's natural urges over attempting to produce a bowel movement 'on schedule.'"*

Managing Difficulties with Bladder Control

Bladder changes in Parkinson's can include **frequency** (needing to urinate often), **urgency** (feeling as if one needs to urinate immediately), or difficulty with fully emptying the bladder. These bladder difficulties sometimes prevent people with Parkinson disease from drinking enough fluids, because they try to avoid a sudden need to use the bathroom. Remember to drink fluids throughout the day, even if not feeling thirsty. Some people find it helpful to limit their fluid intake in the evening hours to prevent frequent nighttime trips to the bathroom. Individuals with both bladder urgency and mobility problems may wish to consider obtaining a urinal or bedside commode for nighttime use.

Another reason that some people have to get up in the night to use the bathroom is that they have ankle swelling. All the fluid that accumulates in the feet and ankles throughout the day reenters the circulation once the person is reclining, and the kidneys try to rid the body of the extra fluid by producing more urine. If this is a problem, then medications to reduce swelling, the use of elastic stockings, or simply elevating the legs in the evening a few hours before bedtime may reduce the nocturnal frequency.

Speak with your physician about any bladder problems you are experiencing. Sometimes medications can be helpful (see also Chapter 7). Developing a regular schedule for toileting may also help with bladder control. Choosing clothing that is easy to remove in the bathroom (such as garments with elastic waistbands and without complex fasteners or belts), use of incontinence pads, or both may help reduce stress and frustration about getting to the bathroom promptly.

Dealing with Loss of Mobility in the Advanced Stages

Individuals living with advanced-stage Parkinson's may experience significant limitations in mobility. It is important to maintain a regular schedule for changing positions throughout the day and night to maintain adequate circulation and skin integrity. Try to change position at least every hour during the waking day and every two to three hours at night. A caregiver may need to provide assistance with these position changes. Use of pillows or cushions can help one maintain a comfortable position and good body alignment. Rubbing skin with lotion or oil can also help circulation and prevent redness or pressure areas.

If mobility changes make regular walking difficult, a wheelchair may be needed for transport around the home or community. Make sure the wheelchair is fitted properly for the user's height and body size, and obtain a cushion for the seat, back, or both to maintain proper positioning in the chair.

Dealing with Mild Cognitive Symptoms

Some people with Parkinson disease experience changes in concentration, memory, or processing of information. These changes, though not always severe, can be frustrating in daily life. A calm environment free of distractions can help a person with such difficulties to focus attention on the task at hand. Multitasking and multiple-step processes (such as following a dessert-baking recipe) can be especially challenging for persons living with Parkinson disease. It is important to create an environment that will allow concentration on the task at hand. Needless to say, distractions during driving can have dire consequences for anyone, but particularly so for people with Parkinson's.

Keep eyeglasses, keys, and other regularly used items in consistent "assigned places" to prevent hunting for lost or misplaced items. Countless people with Parkinson disease have fallen and injured themselves while frantically looking for their keys, coat, and other items when running late for an appointment. Many people find it helpful to keep a calendar of appointments and events as a memory aid for their scheduled activities. Practicing trivia, crossword puzzles, Sudoku, or other "neurobics" games can help keep your thinking skills sharp.

Managing Confusion, Hallucinations, and Dementia

If thinking changes become more severe, it is important to take steps to ensure the individual's safety and comfort. To prevent confusion, caregivers can help create an environment free of clutter or unneeded items. Remove medications or small items that could be mistaken as food items from places the person with Parkinson's can reach. Installing safety latches on basement doors or cupboards containing hazardous products can help prevent accidents.

It is not usually advisable to argue with someone who has dementia or hallucinations, as it can result in escalating confusion or agitation. Try to maintain a calm environment, keeping your voice volume low. It can sometimes help to distract the person by changing the subject, offering a rest period, providing a snack, or suggesting an alternative activity. Care partners should plan for increased confusion or even agitation with any change in their loved one's environment, such as taking a trip, staying at an unfamiliar place, or moving into a new living environment.

Rapid changes in thinking can be the result of illness, infection, or injury. Bladder infections, which may occur without any alarming symptoms, are notorious for causing sudden changes in the mental function of persons with Parkinson's and dementia. Some medications can also cause confusion or hallucinations as a side effect. Caregivers should consult the patient's physician if they observe sudden thinking changes.

Dealing with Apathy, Depression, Impulsivity, and Anxiety

Many symptoms related to Parkinson's involve a person's emotional world. Changes in mood and personality can occur. Some patients develop apathy: the loss of interest, motivation, and initiative. This may result in a decreased desire to participate in activities the person enjoyed in the past or a tendency to sit passively for extended periods. Encourage the person to exercise and engage in other activity throughout the day. Even short periods of movement help to improve circulation, reduce muscle stiffness, and maintain motor function. A care partner often has to take the initiative. Parkinson's patients who experience apathy will still enjoy their favorite activities once someone else "gets them going."

Depression is often seen in Parkinson's and is related to the chemical imbalance in the brain. It is important to address feelings of depression or note changes in sleep patterns, appetite, or mood with your physician. Many people with Parkinson's benefit from prescribed antidepressant medications. Others find counseling, exercise, support groups, or other activities to be helpful in coping with depression. A combination of many strategies is usually the most effective management. Care partners need to be on the alert for signs of depression in the person with Parkinson's. Any suicidal thoughts should trigger an immediate call to the person's physician or to a crisis-consulting agency. Be aware that the risk of suicide may be somewhat higher for the first few weeks of treatment with certain antidepressants, as well as after deep-brain stimulation surgery. Such instances require increased vigilance on the part of the care partner.

Impulsive behaviors (trying to move too quickly or engage in unsafe behaviors like climbing and overreaching) are sometimes seen in Parkinson disease. Impulse-control disorders (compulsive gambling, eating, or shopping; hypersexuality) have been linked to the use of some dopamine agonist medications. Make sure to discuss any impulsive or compulsive behaviors with your physician, even if the activity does not seem harmful (such as cleaning or rearranging furniture). Medication adjustments may be warranted.

It is estimated that approximately 40 percent of people with Parkinson's experience anxiety. This can range from a mild anxiety disorder to panic attacks and is sometimes linked to the person's medication schedules or wearing off. Medications and counseling can be helpful in managing anxiety. Other activities such as deep breathing, biofeedback, meditation, tai chi, and yoga are sometimes helpful. Make sure to report any feelings of anxiety to your treating physician or health care provider for recommendations most suitable to your situation.

Managing Sleep Changes in Parkinson Disease

Many factors contribute a restful night's sleep. Parkinson disease can interrupt the sleep cycle at both ends of the spectrum, creating insomnia for some people and drowsiness for others. Medication side effects can worsen sleep changes by causing excessive sleepiness or frightening nightmares. Practical strategies to help ensure good rest include the following:

- Try to stay on a regular schedule, keeping bedtime consistent.
- Get adequate exercise.
- Avoid excessive daytime sleeping.
- Limit fluid intake after 7 p.m. if bladder changes result in frequent nighttime trips to the bathroom.
- Use satin-based nightwear or a "slippery fabric" drawsheet in the middle third of the bed to make rolling and getting up from bed easier.

- Use a lightweight comforter to avoid having multiple sheets and blankets, which can get tangled up with your feet and restrict bed mobility.
- Keep the bedroom at a comfortable temperature for sleeping.
- Seek a referral to physical or occupational therapy for advice on safe and comfortable positioning and techniques for getting in and out of bed more easily.
- Contact your physician for advice on medication adjustments if immobility prevents you from rolling in bed or getting into bed safely at night.
- Report feelings of restless legs, frequent nightmares, or "acting out" dreams to your physician.

Managing Orthostatic Hypotension

Orthostatic hypotension—low blood pressure made worse by rising from a chair or bed—can occur in people with Parkinson disease. This can lead to feelings of dizziness, vision changes, difficulty thinking clearly, or fainting or loss of consciousness. Falls can also occur. The following actions can help deal with orthostatic hypotension:

- Have your blood pressure checked in both seated and standing positions.
- Avoid rapid position changes. Sit on the edge of the bed before getting up. Stand for a moment after rising from a chair to make sure you are not feeling dizzy.
- Maintain adequate fluid intake. Dehydration can cause even larger drops in standing blood pressure.
- Consider when dizziness or fainting episodes occur. Many people notice increased difficulty immediately after eating a full meal, when their digestive system requires increased blood flow. If these episodes are worse after meals, consider eating smaller, more frequent meals during the day.

- After being seated for longer periods, move your arms and legs around to stimulate circulation before getting up.
- Seek advice from your physician, nurse, or dietitian about increasing your salt intake, which may help keep blood pressure from dropping.
- Wearing elastic support stockings is sometimes helpful, but they may be difficult to put on and wear regularly. Ask your medical team members for their input and recommendations.
- Some people benefit from the use of medications to keep standing blood pressure at higher levels.

Weight Loss

Medication effects, difficulty swallowing, depression, and other medical factors can contribute to weight loss in people with Parkinson's. If unexpected or unwanted weight loss occurs, include calorie-dense foods at mealtime and eat between-meal snacks, liquid supplements, or both. Remember that slowed movements can affect chewing and swallowing and may cause someone to fatigue before finishing a meal. Parkinson disease causes the stomach to move—and therefore empty—more slowly, which can cause a feeling of fullness early in the meal, a condition called early satiety. Try smaller, more frequent meals if fatigue or early satiety becomes an issue. Seek a referral to occupational therapy if you are having difficulty with the mechanics of eating, such as managing silverware and cutting food. Vision changes in contrast sensitivity may make it more difficult to see food on the plate. Use color-contrasting dishes when possible to compensate for these visual changes. Your physician, nurse, or dietitian can provide additional recommendations. Swallowing difficulties should be assessed by a licensed speech pathologist. In the end stages of the disease, maintaining proper nutrition may require the placement of a gastrostomy tube (see also earlier in this chapter under "Managing Swallowing Problems"). If weight loss occurs despite adequate nutrient intake, it's very important to consult with your general practitioner or internist to look for other possible causes.

Keeping Skin in Shape

People with Parkinson's may experience increased redness, flakiness, or irritation of their skin. This is called seborrheic dermatitis, and is more prominent around the nose, eyebrows, and forehead. Although it is rarely a serious problem, the following tips will help keep seborrheic dermatitis under control:

- Wash affected areas daily using a mild, bland soap such as Basis, Dove, or Ivory. Rub gently.
- Apply 1-percent hydrocortisone cream (available over the counter at drugstores) sparingly to affected areas.
- Mild astringents such as witch hazel can be used to reduce oiliness.
- Control dandruff or flaky scalp with shampoos that contain selenium (such as Tegrin or Neutrogena T/Gel).

People with Parkinson disease have an increased risk for melanoma (a dangerous form of skin cancer). Check your skin regularly for any changes. Avoid too much sun, particularly between 10 a.m. and 2 p.m. and in midsummer. Sunlamps and tanning beds should also be avoided. Use a sunscreen with an SPF (sun protection factor) of 15 or higher, even on cloudy days. Apply the sunscreen thoroughly to all exposed skin, including around the eyes, ears, and mouth and on any areas on your head that are bald or have thinning hair. Ultraviolet (UV) rays can penetrate through loosely woven clothing, so wear sunscreen even on areas covered by clothes. Apply non-oil-based moisturizing lotion after a bath or shower. A lip balm with the sunscreen para-aminobenzoic acid (PABA) and UV-opaque sunglasses are also recommended.

Hospitalization

Health changes or injury may result in a hospital stay. Parkinson disease symptoms may escalate during periods of illness or injury, so many people require more assistance than usual for general mobility. Hospital medications are often given on set schedules different from what the person with Parkinson disease is used to, compromising mobility further. Bed rest may increase feelings of stiffness and muscle rigidity. Hospital staff may not be familiar with Parkinson's or the unique needs of the Parkinson's patient.

Make sure you carry a detailed listing of your medication schedule with you, and advocate with the hospital for receiving your medications according to this timetable. Ask your attending physician to write specific orders about the importance of medication timing. Even after doing these things, difficulties may still occur, as hospital schedules are not usually set up to accommodate special requests or timetables. A family care partner may need to advocate for a person with Parkinson disease who is ill or injured. Some hospital settings will allow the patient or care partner to assume responsibility for administering Parkinson disease medications.

Health professionals unfamiliar with Parkinson's may not fully understand motor fluctuations or changes in a person's ability to walk, eat, or dress through the course of the day. Reinforce with the hospital staff the concept that some people with Parkinson disease move differently at certain times of the day, and let the staff know that you may need more assistance during "off periods." Do not hesitate to ask your attending physician to consult with your neurologist, who may be able to give additional information about your overall health history as well as provide useful advice about needed medication changes, drugs that should be avoided, and so forth.

Try to get up and start moving as soon as possible during the hospital stay, but always with your treating physician's consent. Seek a referral to physical therapy to provide bedside exercise assistance if you are unable to get up, and ask to begin a course of rehabilitation therapies prior to discharge to restore flexibility, strength, and endurance. For more prolonged hospitalizations, a period of inpatient rehabilitation at a specialized facility may be necessary.

Elective Surgery

In deciding whether or not undergo elective surgery (such as joint replacement and cosmetic procedures), it is important to carefully consider the potential impact of Parkinson disease. Seek input from your neurologist or movement disorder specialist to discuss your plans and receive appropriate recommendations.

Most surgeries will cause an interruption in your medication schedule. Make sure the surgeon is aware that you have Parkinson disease and will need your medications resumed as soon as possible following surgery. Some surgical procedures may allow you to take your Parkinson disease medications with a sip of water even on the morning of surgery, but you must receive clearance from the surgeon prior to doing so. Some anti-Parkinson medications may not mix well with certain anesthetics, and your surgeon may ask you to stop them weeks in advance. In such instances always check if that is safe to do with your neurologist, as some of these medications should not be discontinued abruptly. There is a long list of medications that persons with Parkinson disease should not take because they may make their symptoms worse. Unfortunately, with the standardization of procedures at hospitals, orders for such medications may be entered automatically. Therefore always be aware, to the best of your ability, of what medicines you are given and for what reason. For example, many nausea medications and tranquilizers should be avoided in persons with Parkinson's.

As your body undergoes the stress of recovery, be aware that it often takes longer for people with Parkinson disease to resume a normal routine after surgery. Follow-up rehabilitation therapies can help restore function, whether provided at home, in a transitional-care setting, or on an outpatient basis. It is important to remain as active as possible within recommended restriction guidelines. Don't forget the importance of good nutrition and adequate rest throughout the recovery process.

Medications to Avoid

Medications that block the action of dopamine should not be given to persons with Parkinson disease unless they have been shown to not worsen the symptoms of the disease or unless they are absolutely necessary. Such medications are called antidopaminergic drugs and are used mainly to treat nausea, slow stomach movement, and psychotic symptoms such as hallucinations and paranoia. Some common antipsychotics are haloperidol (Haldol), chlorpromazine (Thorazine), and risperidone (Risperidal). An antidopaminergic medication often used for stomach trouble is metoclopramide (Reglan). Many antinausea medications, such as prochlorperazine (Compazine), trimethobenzamide (Tigan), and promethazine (Phenergan)—this last one (also used as an antihistamine), work through blocking dopamine actions and can worsen the symptoms of Parkinson disease. Always check with your doctor and your pharmacist whether it's OK to take any newly prescribed drug with your Parkinson's.

Chapter 10

Lifestyle Changes and Disease Management

The Importance of Exercise

Michael is an active 44-year-old man who has been living with Parkinson disease for four years. He loves to run for exercise and fun. Since his diagnosis, he has continued to run about two miles a day, performing regular warm-up stretching before hitting the streets. Sometimes, Michael experiences dystonia (painful muscle cramping and abnormal foot posturing) while running. As a result, he's adjusted his schedule to exercise at times he feels his medication is working best.

Susan is a 57-year-old woman who has been living with Parkinson's for three years. She works full-time as a billing clerk at a local hospital. Because she's tired after work, Susan has adjusted her schedule in order to go for a 30-minute walk before heading in to the office. She also uses a yoga DVD at home several times a week and feels that regular stretching provides her with the greatest benefit in reducing her feelings of muscle stiffness. At work, she performs brief stretches she learned in physical therapy to combat neck and shoulder stiffness.

Paul is a 70-year-old man who has been diagnosed with Parkinson's for seven years. Although retired, he maintains an active lifestyle and enjoys travel, gardening, and golf. Paul attends a local health club three or four days per week, where he uses the strength-training machines, treadmill, and stationary bike. Paul gets advice from a personal trainer at the club. He finds this keeps him motivated to exercise.

Irene is an 82-year-old woman who has been living with Parkinson disease for 15 years. She recently completed physical therapy treatment and is following through with a home exercise program designed to work on her flexibility, leg strength, balance, and walking skills. Irene spends approximately an hour each day working on these activities, focusing on making large, exaggerated motions while exercising. Her husband provides her with support and assistance as needed. Irene has also begun to participate in an exercise group twice a week at a local Parkinson's center.

> **Exercise** is an important component of an integrated treatment plan for Parkinson disease.

Although the individuals described above are quite different, they have all taken steps to incorporate exercise into their routine. Exercise is recommended as part of a fully integrated treatment program for people with Parkinson's. The benefits of exercise are many and include improved strength, bone health, flexibility, and endurance. Recent studies suggest that exercise may have a disease-modifying effect on Parkinson's by helping remaining dopamine cells to function more efficiently. Research has also suggested that for Parkinson's patients to receive maximal benefits, exercise must challenge the individual by being specific, intense, and repetitive. (See more on exercise in Chapter 7).

Here are several tips to consider with respect to exercising with Parkinson disease:

- Take your general health into account when planning your exercise program. Consider any condition or past injury that could be aggravated by increased activity, and check with your physician regarding the appropriateness of your planned program.

- Set realistic goals, creating an exercise program that fits into your schedule and budget. Setting a regular time for exercise each day will help you adhere to your routine. Every person is different, but it is often helpful to choose a time to exercise when you are usually functioning well and are not too tired.
- Make sure you include activities that promote flexibility, strength, balance, and cardiovascular conditioning in your routine. Exercises promoting trunk flexibility are very important, even in early stages of the disease. Exercises designed to improve core strength (abdominal and trunk muscles) are also recommended. Consider programs such as tai chi or yoga, which offer an integrated approach that promotes stretching, strengthening, and balance training. In addition to the usual exercise benefits, a walking program gives you an opportunity to improve your walking pattern: you can try to focus on large steps and wide turns while walking.
- If balance changes make standing or walking exercises unsafe, design your program so that you do most exercises while lying down or sitting. Maintaining a good general activity level is also important. Gardening, yard work, golf, tennis, and household chores all provide some contribution to the overall value of exercise, but they cannot substitute for a structured exercise program.
- Contact a physical therapist or an exercise physiologist for an evaluation and assistance in developing an appropriate exercise program. Membership in a local health club may offer access to equipment and skilled staff who can provide guidance. Joining a community exercise class or group sponsored by a health facility or senior center can also help you "stick with the program" through the support and encouragement of other class participants.

**Ask the Experts: I Have Been Diagnosed with Parkinson's.
What Should I Watch or Change in My Diet?**

Susan Imke, GNP-C, says: "A frequent question asked by those living with Parkinson disease is 'Should I be following a special diet?' In general, people are encouraged to eat a balanced diet, with foods from all four basic food groups (fruits and vegetables, grains, meats, and dairy). A healthy diet usually limits red meat and avoids foods high in salt, processed sugar, and saturated fats. Many dietitians recommend augmenting a well-balanced diet with daily vitamin and mineral supplements as a nutritional 'insurance policy,' taking these supplements with food. It is not advised to choose a megadose vitamin formula.

"There is growing evidence that foods rich in antioxidants may have health benefits for everyone, including people with Parkinson disease. Many antioxidant supplements purchased without a prescription do not affect brain health, because they are unable to cross the protective blood–brain barrier. Natural antioxidants found in foods are able to enter the brain and are most plentiful in foods such as fruits and vegetables, walnuts, green tea, grape juice, red wine, and dark chocolate.

"Medications used to treat the symptoms of Parkinson disease may be affected by when and what types of food are eaten. Proteins found in food compete with levodopa for absorption in the stomach and small intestine. So it's best to take levodopa on an empty stomach. Four or five ounces of nondairy fluid taken with the levodopa tablet prior to eating (even 15 minutes before may be enough) will propel the drug faster through the stomach and into the small intestine, where it will get absorbed into the bloodstream. Think of it as giving the levodopa a head start on absorption over the food about to be eaten.

(Continued)

(Continued)

"Typically the people most affected by protein are those who experience significant on/off motor fluctuations, who take levodopa four or more times per day, or both. To verify if protein is interfering with levodopa absorption, experiment with a vegetarian diet or move the daily recommended allotment of protein to the evening meal. Altering the timing of protein intake may help prevent interference with levodopa absorption. Reducing overall amounts of daily protein may also prove helpful, but note that protein is important to overall nutrition and that even those people who are 'protein sensitive' should not try to eliminate protein from their diet. It is advisable to avoid taking levodopa-containing medications with milk, yogurt, pudding, or other protein-rich foods. Consult with your physician to see if other dietary changes are advisable. Referral to a nurse or a licensed dietitian familiar with Parkinson disease for additional recommendations may also be helpful.

"Nausea can occur as a side effect of medications. If levodopa causes nausea, a small cracker or bite of fruit can be taken with doses required between meals. Pretzels are excellent, because they require no refrigeration. Crystallized ginger can be nibbled to offset nausea.

"Parkinson disease may affect the ability to eat and digest food efficiently. Just as it causes slowness in movement, Parkinson's also slows gastric (gut) motility. In Parkinson's patients, chewing and swallowing may be prolonged, stomach emptying may be delayed, and food moves through the intestines more slowly relative to someone who does not have the disease. For all these reasons, nutrients may be better absorbed when the person with Parkinson's eats small amounts frequently rather than three large meals per day.

"As eating and digestive processes slow down, weight loss can become a problem for many people who have Parkinson's.

(Continued)

(Continued)

Frequent, small meals can help them to maintain optimal weight. Liquid supplements can be useful. Sometimes patients are so diligent in limiting fat intake and worrying about protein restrictions that they deprive themselves of much-needed calories.

"Maintaining adequate fluid intake may become more difficult for people who have difficulty swallowing or who are reluctant to drink liquids because of bladder changes sometimes seen in Parkinson's. Our natural sense of thirst may diminish with age, and anti-Parkinson drugs also dry out the body. It is important to drink water 'by the clock,' not unlike the way one schedules crucial medications. This allows better absorption of nutrients from foods as well as of medications and reduces the risk of dehydration."

Leisure Activities

Generally, it is important to stay active when living with Parkinson's. Recreational activities provide physical, mental, and social stimulation as well as keep us connected with friends and family. Keep your physician and other team members informed if you have experienced significant changes in your pursuit of leisure interests because of mobility challenges, depression, or anxiety.

Many people with Parkinson's report that they feel at their best when engaged in activities they truly enjoy. Hobbies and leisure interests promote relaxation and are essential to replenish mind, body, and spirit. It is wise to make a commitment to ensure adequate time for leisure pursuits within your regular schedule. Although Parkinson disease can change involvement in past interests, simple adaptations may allow continued enjoyment of leisure activities. For example, avid gardeners may wish to consider installing raised flower beds to improve access to their garden space, and cyclists may want to try using a recumbent bike to continue riding.

Remember that Parkinson's often makes movement slower and can affect balance. To ensure safety, proceed cautiously when attempting activities you have not performed in some time. Remember that warm-up stretches help prepare stiff and rigid muscles for activity. Be mindful that fatigue or "off time" also affects your ability to fully engage in more active leisure pursuits. Remember to take medications with you and keep taking pills on schedule.

Changes caused by the disease also create opportunities to try new leisure interests. Exploring new activities promotes creative expression and enhances quality of life. Many people have been pleasantly surprised to discover a hidden talent for creative outlets like painting, writing, sculpting, or photography that was unrecognized before their diagnosis of Parkinson disease.

Stress Management

We live in a world of schedules, deadlines, and multitasking that often increase stress levels. Most people with Parkinson's find that physical and emotional stressors often make their symptoms worse. When under stress, they may experience increased tremor, slowness, or other symptoms when fighting a cold or flu. Some patients note increased difficulty with Parkinson's symptoms if they feel worried, anxious, or upset. To help reduce stress, here are strategies some people with Parkinson disease are using:

- **Judy, age 62:** "Placing all my appointments and commitments on one calendar reduces chances of overbooking my schedule. I schedule my 'rest breaks' too!"

- **Michelle, age 57:** "I have revised my wardrobe to get rid of blouses with small buttons, jewelry with small clasps, and other items, to make my morning routine flow more smoothly."
- **Jose, age 68:** "I fill out the check blanks with most of the necessary information before leaving home, to reduce stress when standing in a line of people at the grocery store."
- **Gary, age 47:** "I give myself extra time to get out the door for work, church services, or scheduled appointments, to reduce feeling hurried or rushed."
- **Sadie, age 72:** "I have finally learned to say 'no.' It's a simple word, but often difficult to say. Agreeing to too many commitments builds stress in my daily life."

Some people with Parkinson's find it helpful to schedule time for relaxation each day. Simple deep-breathing exercises can reduce stress and promote relaxation. Use of soft music or relaxation tapes can also prove helpful. Massage, active exercise, and meditation are also used by many to combat stress levels.

Persons living with Parkinson disease often experience anxiety disorders. Significant feelings of unmanageable stress, anxiety, or panic should be discussed with a physician. He or she can assess the need for treatment with medications and make referrals to a social service agency or a mental health professional. (More information on anxiety can be found in Chapters 4, 7, and 9.)

Driving

Depending on where you live, the ability to drive may be an important part of daily life. Slowed movements, vision changes, neck stiffness, and difficulty with multitasking caused by Parkinson disease can all have a negative impact on safe driving. Here are tips to make driving easier:

- Alter your driving schedule to avoid peak traffic and times when your medications are not working well.
- Reduce night driving if Parkinson's is affecting your vision in low-light settings. A 2009 study published in *Neurology* found that compared with the general population, Parkinson's patients have double the risk of automobile accidents when driving in fog or low light.
- Because people with Parkinson's can have difficulty with multitasking, focus your attention on the road by turning off the radio, not talking on your cell phone, and avoiding other distractions.
- Get out of the car frequently to stretch and move around. Remember to stretch your neck and shoulder muscles too.
- Make sure your car seat offers good support or obtain a support cushion for improved posture and driving comfort.

The time may come when the ability to drive safely becomes too compromised by Parkinson's symptoms. Each person must maintain honest self-assessment or obtain feedback from trusted friends or family members on whether it's still safe to drive. For more-formalized assessment, seek a referral to an occupational therapist who can perform a driving evaluation and offer recommendations for changes or modifications.

It is wise to plan ahead and consider alternative transportation for when driving independently is no longer an option. Car pools or public transportation may be options for some people. Others may need to make arrangements for rides from friends, neighbors, and family members. Some communities have volunteers who will driver patients to medical appointments, grocery shopping, and other errands. In addition, many religious entities (such as churches, synagogues, and mosques) help arrange rides to attend religious services.

Using Complementary Therapies

Many people with Parkinson disease choose to explore the use of complementary or alternative therapies. While there is still a substantial lack of evidence-based research in this area indicating clear benefits, many people try acupuncture, massage, and a variety of other complementary options for overall health and wellness. One study suggested that less than one-half of people with Parkinson's who use complementary therapies report them to their physician. It is always preferable to openly discuss all treatments you are using with your health care providers, to ensure they have a full understanding of all aspects of your health.

Spirituality

Living well with Parkinson's requires attention to mind, body, and spirit. The diagnosis of Parkinson's affects plans and dreams for the future. This altered path can contribute to feelings of bewilderment, anger, and sadness. It is important to acknowledge these feelings and grieve the associated losses. Many people turn to their spiritual beliefs to help make sense of their feelings and emotions. It is normal to ask "Why me?" or to seek a higher power to help deal with this unforeseen event. Sorting out your emotions by exploring your beliefs and values is a normal process toward building resiliency and hope.

Hope helps us live with unpredictability and see our situation in a new light. Most organized religions and spiritual beliefs are built on a foundation of hope. Even people with advanced symptoms of Parkinson disease single out feelings of hope as a powerful tool in coping with the challenges of everyday life. Some studies have cited a connection between prayer and health outcomes.

Not all people view spirituality as being connected with organized religion. A connection to nature, keeping a journal, meditation, and use of inner resources such as optimism, humor, and motivation can all be manifestations of spirituality and may be powerful supports when one is living with Parkinson disease.

Travel

Whether it is related to business or pleasure or is frequent or rare, it is likely that people with Parkinson's will want to travel. However, travel plans may need to be changed to accommodate challenges caused by Parkinson's. It is advisable to choose your itinerary wisely. Ask questions before you start. It's important to conduct research on the area to which you will be traveling, on accessibility issues, and on time schedules for the trip. Itineraries that provide flexibility, luggage assistance, and easy-to-negotiate surroundings may be best. If necessary, find a travel agent who is willing to work with you to design an ideal travel experience. If you want to have grab bars, accessible showers, and raised toilet seats available, make an advance request for accessible hotel accommodations or cruise cabins. Schedule time for rest as needed. Take an extra day on arrival or before departure to rest before you set out on your travels, or arrange to stop along the way for a refreshing break.

Make sure new luggage purchases are lightweight and have wheels. When flying, remember to keep medications in carry-on luggage, not in a checked suitcase. It is advisable to carry extra medication with you in case of travel delays. Minimize your luggage, but make sure you take items that are necessary for a good travel experience. If you sometimes use a cane or walker, take it with you. This advice is sometimes ignored but shouldn't be. So we'll say it again: if you sometimes use a cane or walker, take it with you.

Change position frequently when traveling. When driving long distances, stop every hour or so for a brief stretch. When flying, perform shoulder shrugs, ankle circles, and neck and arm motions.

If flying, you may wish to request an aisle or bulkhead seat to allow for extra legroom. To decrease travel stress, use skycaps, airport wheelchair assistance, and luggage porters. If possible, avoid checking wheelchairs or walkers. If traveling with a wheelchair, walker, or cane, keep it with you until you arrive at the flight gate for boarding, and request that it be returned to you as soon as you get off the plane. Take advantage of calls for preboarding to give yourself extra time. If your medications need to be given by injection (for example, apomorphine), you may need a note from your doctor to be allowed to carry the necessary supplies on board with you.

Being outside your normal living environment can sometimes prove disruptive. Consider any time changes within your itinerary to adjust your medication schedule accordingly. You may need to improvise if you normally use adaptive equipment to make daily life easier. For example, a straight-back chair against the side of the bed can serve as a makeshift bed-rail assist.

It is wise to ask for advice and help when needed. Hotel concierges, cruise pursers' desks, and Chamber of Commerce travel information stops can provide information and assistance for persons with physical mobility challenges. Above all, try to have fun! Travel can be an adventure, even if it is common to experience delays and disruptions in routine.

The Power of Music and Dance

Music and rhythm have been shown to have an impact on the nervous system. We are all aware that certain types of music raise our spirits and make us want to move, while others help us relax and unwind at the end of a long day. Research in music therapy for Parkinson's has demonstrated that moving to music can help an individual achieve better range of motion, improve walking cadence, and reduce freezing. Use of a metronome or music with a steady beat provides a backdrop to help "set the pace" and keep people with Parkinson's moving more easily.

Music also evokes beneficial emotional responses. Creative musical activities such as improvisation, drumming, songwriting, and discussion of lyrics have been used successfully to help individuals express their thoughts and emotions, reduce stress, and find a sense of accomplishment.

Several studies have recently been published indicating the benefits of dance in people with Parkinson disease. Individuals participating in twice-weekly dance classes showed improvements in balance, functional mobility, and walking. Active exercise combined with the benefits of enhanced movement through music and rhythm is the suggested basis for such improvements.

Music therapists are trained professionals who offer therapeutic interventions to restore, maintain, or improve function using music. Neurological music therapy is a type of music therapy specialized for treating neurologic patients. Neurological music therapists work in a variety of care settings, though they may not be as common as other therapists on an interdisciplinary team. In many states, music therapy is not eligible for insurance reimbursement. To find a music therapist in your area, visit the American Music Therapy Association website at www.musictherapy.org.

Getting Involved in the Parkinson's Community

Meeting other people with Parkinson's and sharing common concerns in a support group setting can be very helpful. There are a number of online and in-person support groups available. Some groups are geared more for the recently diagnosed or those with young-onset

Parkinson's. It is usually best to do some initial investigation so that you can find out more about a group's goals, its format, and who usually attends before deciding if it will be a good fit for you.

There are also opportunities for involvement in Parkinson's research studies. These can take the form of surveys, medication trials, interviews, or other types of participation. It is important to ask questions regarding the study's design, along with any potential benefits or risks, before deciding to participate. Your physician may be aware of research studies in your area, or you can investigate a number of ongoing studies at www.pdtrials.org. (There's more on research in Chapter 11.)

Some people with Parkinson disease choose to become involved through advocacy, fund-raising, or volunteerism. Many people feel that a sense of involvement in such activities contributes to overall quality of life. Contact a local or national Parkinson's center or organization to learn more.

Although there are a variety of ways to become involved in Parkinson-related activities, each individual must decide her or his own level of interest and comfort in doing so. Some people find it upsetting to be involved in activities where other people with Parkinson's may be in a more advanced stage of the disease. Some are not comfortable sharing their thoughts and feelings in a group setting. There is no right or wrong decision on getting involved; the decision is yours. (There is more information on community involvement and advocacy in Chapter 13.)

Ask the Experts: How Should I Prepare for Doctor's Appointments?

Susan Imke, GNP-C, has the following advice:
- *"Choose your health care providers carefully. You should feel confident in their knowledge and understanding of Parkinson*

(Continued)

(*Continued*)

disease. You should feel comfortable asking questions. You should feel like your concerns are being addressed. If possible, seek care in a Parkinson's specialty clinic.

- "Try to arrive to scheduled appointments a few minutes early, giving yourself adequate time to complete the check-in process and any paperwork.
- "Take a current list of medications with you to all medical appointments. Include the medication names, dosages, and timing schedules. This is particularly important in a new care setting or an emergency room.
- "Take someone with you to neurology appointments to share observations that supplement your own report and to listen carefully to the advice or directions you are given.
- "Think about priorities for your appointment beforehand, and jot down questions so you'll remember to ask them. If your list is long, be aware that you may not be able to discuss every issue and that you may need to make a follow-up appointment.
- "Be your own best advocate! Your physician is a capable coach of your health care team, but you are the owner. Familiarize yourself with the role of all team members, such as rehabilitation therapists, social workers, and nurses. Seek referrals to other professionals as questions or problems arise.
- "Make sure you understand all instructions prior to leaving your appointment. Ask questions if instructions are unclear.
- "Provide necessary information to ensure that reports are sent to your other physicians and health care team members. Sign the necessary medical release forms, and have complete names, addresses, and phone numbers of these health care team members readily accessible.

(*Continued*)

(*Continued*)

- "*Keep telephone reports brief and to the point, and when possible, speak for yourself.*
- "*If you need to be admitted to a hospital, transitional-care setting, or nursing home, be aware that many of the staff are unlikely to have special expertise in Parkinson disease. Your medication schedules are likely to be disrupted. Be prepared to provide information or answer the same questions repeatedly. Caregivers may need to step in to advocate for someone with a recent illness or injury.*"

More on choosing your doctor and the roles of the members of your health care team can be found in Chapter 5.

Chapter 11

Research

For most people living with Parkinson disease, research represents the hope of a cure, and this hope is what often triggers a desire to participate in experimental trials. Before deciding to become a volunteer for Parkinson disease research it is important to learn about the types of research studies that may be available. It is equally important to understand one's own reasons for agreeing to participate in research and realize that there may be risks, both evident and hidden, associated with such decisions. In this chapter we will provide some basic information about research that will hopefully answer some of the most frequent questions and concerns that surround decisions whether or not to take part in research.

Why Should I Consider Participating in Research?

People with chronic illnesses are often drawn to research because they hope that research will give them a chance to receive newer, better treatments or maybe even a cure. Although hope is a good thing, this is probably the wrong reason to become a volunteer for research. The word "volunteer" here is used intentionally: becoming a research participant or a research subject, as studies often refer to participants, is an act of volunteering. The best reason for participating in research is a desire to help science progress toward better treatments and eventually a cure. Without volunteers research cannot progress, and 10 or 20 years from now people with Parkinson's and doctors who treat them will not be any more effective than they are today. There is only one thing that can change this, and that's research.

At the center of the research effort stand the many people with Parkinson disease who volunteer to become subjects. Although volunteering may sound too altruistic, participating in research does often provide some "fringe benefits." For one, it gives a person with Parkinson disease the opportunity to fight back. The research volunteer becomes a soldier of an army fighting for the cure. Just as in a war, battles may be won or lost, but what motivates the fight is the hope for the final victory, even though it may take years to get there. Besides this "feel good" benefit, participating in research usually involves receiving very detailed evaluations and tests, which may discover and result in the treatment of other, unsuspected health problems.

Volunteering to participate in research helps improve our understanding and treatment of Parkinson's.

Consider an illustrative example: Albert was in his late 40s and had just been diagnosed with Parkinson disease when he agreed to participate in a placebo-controlled (this term is explained later in this chapter) research trial of a new medication that had shown promise for slowing the progression of the disease. As part of the screening tests he had to see a dermatologist (skin specialist) for an examination. The dermatologist had bad and good news for Albert. She pointed out a small dark spot on Albert's back, which he and his family physician had never noticed before. She told Albert that this was likely a melanoma, a form of skin cancer that can be life-threatening if not treated in the early stages. The dermatologist took out the lesion, which indeed turned out to be a melanoma, and reassured Albert that the cancer had been detected and treated early enough to not be a cause of concern anymore. Albert was unable to be part of the research study, but his decision to volunteer to do so may have saved his life.

What Kinds of Research Studies May Be Open to a Person with Parkinson Disease?

Generally speaking, there are two types of research studies in which you may be able to participate. The first type does not involve investigating a form of treatment. Studies of this sort are usually **observational**, and their aim is to better understand the symptoms of Parkinson disease, the development and evolution of such symptoms over time, and the risk factors leading to such symptoms. Observational studies also look into the possible causes, genetic or environmental, of the disease. The second type of study is called **interventional**. Such studies evaluate the potential benefit of an "intervention," be that a new drug, therapy, or surgery.

Observational Studies

Here are some examples of observational studies:

- A scientist (in this case an epidemiologist) wishes to find out if caffeine consumption decreases the risk for Parkinson's. He may design a questionnaire to figure out how much caffeine a person has consumed in the last five years. He will then administer this questionnaire to a group of people with Parkinson's and a group of people without Parkinson's,and compare the results.
- Another scientist may want to take this question a step further and study whether caffeine consumption has any impact on how fast the disease progresses. This scientist may ask

persons living with Parkinson's to record all the forms of caffeine they consume over, say, five years, and in the end see whether the rate of progression correlates with the amount of caffeine consumed.

Similar observational studies may look into how genetics, family history, amount and type of exercise, lifestyle, other health problems, or even socioeconomic factors may influence the risk for developing Parkinson disease, the rate at which the disease progresses, or the types of symptoms that a person develops once they get the disease. The goal of such research, besides trying to predict how some patients may fare compared with others, is to generate ideas about what kinds of changes a person can make to improve her or his own outlook. Such ideas can be further tested with interventional studies (see the next section). One such example would be that if an observational study shows that persons with Parkinson's who exercise regularly do better over the years than the ones who don't, then one could design an interventional study to see if asking patients to exercise alters the course and prognosis of the disease.

Interventional Studies

This second type of research in which persons with Parkinson disease may participate examines the effects of specific treatments— "interventions"—on Parkinson disease. The treatment under study may be a new and promising medication, a new type of surgery, a nutritional supplement, a particular type of therapy or exercise, and so on. The scientists who design such a study specify a hypothesis that they want to test. One such hypothesis, would be, for example, that drug A improves the motor symptoms of Parkinson disease. The scientists also specify the ways that improvement will be measured. In the same example they may decide that the effectiveness of the drug will be measured by comparing patients' scores on the Unified Parkinson's Disease Rating Scale (UPDRS; see Chapter 2) before and after treatment with drug A. They may go as far as specifying that they expect at least, say, a 10% improvement and, based on that expectation, do some statistical calculations to figure out how many persons should participate in the study. (As a rule, a study needs more participants to detect a smaller effect.)

One important aspect of such studies is the **placebo**. It is very well known that when a new treatment is tried, both patients who receive it and doctors who administer it may see improvement in the symptoms even when the new medication is not truly effective. This can even happen when patients are given, say, a pill that contains no medication whatsoever. The word "placebo" refers to such a sham treatment, and the improvement seen with ineffective medications or placebo is called the placebo effect. The placebo effect is a sort of "wishful thinking," and it can be very strong; in fact it has been shown to be fairly strong in Parkinson disease. It is not clear why the placebo effect happens, but it probably has to do with the power of suggestion and the hope created by the simple fact that one is trying something new and promising. Unfortunately, the placebo effect is short-lived, without any long-term benefits. Therefore sham pills are not really useful to treat any diseases.

Because of the placebo effect, most well-designed interventional studies come with two important qualifiers: "placebo-controlled" and "double-blind." The first term means that a portion of the participants will receive a sham intervention, be that a "sugar pill" (it's actually usually a flour pill) or a noneffective form of treatment. For studies of surgical treatments, some participants may actually receive a sham operation! Then the improvement in the group of participants who received the treatment under investigation will be compared to the improvement, if any, in the placebo group. The second qualifier in these studies, "double-blind," means that neither the participants nor the doctors who assess the results of the treatment under study know who receives that treatment and who receives the placebo. This way the doctors can be objective in their assessments, and the "wishful thinking" effect is minimized.

Interventional studies assess not only the effectiveness but also the safety of new treatments. Many of these treatments, particularly medications, have not been used widely, so the full range of their potential unwanted side effects may not be well known. Therefore there may be a risk attached to participating in such studies. For this reason, participants in drug trials usually undergo very extensive medical testing, such as repeated blood tests, electrocardiograms, and urine analysis. Some studies may involve more sophisticated testing, like positron emission tomography (PET) scanning, magnetic resonance imaging (MRI), or a lumbar puncture (also known as a spinal tap). With some studies participants may be asked to provide a sample for analysis of their genes (DNA analysis).

Drug trials of new medications are supervised by the Food and Drug Administration (FDA) in the United States with a very rigorous process to maximize safety and minimize mishaps. Any serious reaction to the medication during the trial must be immediately reported to the drug company that produces the medication and to all the doctors participating in the study. External monitoring committees review all the test results to ensure that no particular patterns of serious complications are emerging as the study progresses. Finally, the physicians who conduct the study are supervised by the institutional review boards (often referred to as the IRBs) of their own institutions. Such multiple levels of supervision and double-checking help ensure not only the validity of the study results but also the well-being of the participants.

Informed Consent

Because of all the concerns mentioned in the previous paragraphs, persons who agree to participate in research have to read and sign an "informed consent" document. This document contains a lot of information about what the study entails, how many visits are required, what kinds of tests will be performed, what potential side effects are already known, and what types of side effects might be possible based on the available scientific knowledge about the particular treatment. For example, an experimental drug may not be known to cause liver damage; however, based on its chemistry, scientists may have reason to believe that it has the potential to cause such damage. In that case frequent testing of liver function may be required by the study design (usually referred to as the study protocol).

It is very important to carefully review the informed consent and have all your questions answered to your satisfaction before signing it. Your signature means that you agree (that is, consent) to participate and that you understand the potential risks and effort involved (that is, you are informed). However, your signature is not a contract, which means that it does not legally bind you in any way. You retain the right to withdraw your consent to participate at any point throughout the study. You will also be given contact information for persons that you may notify if you suspect that the study is not conducted properly. Conversely, the study physician may withdraw you from the study if she or he believes that continuing the study may be detrimental to your health or if your further participation may compromise the scientific integrity of the results (for example, if something happened that convinced your doctor that the diagnosis of Parkinson's was wrong in your case).

Clinical drug studies are classified as Phase 1, 2, 3, or 4 studies. These are the phases of testing the drug in humans after it has already been extensively tested in experimental animals. Phase 1 studies test the safety of the drug and find out the necessary and safe dosage in normal volunteers and persons with the disease of interest—in our case, Parkinson's. Phase 2 studies focus on drug safety in a small number of persons with Parkinson's while also assessing the drug's effectiveness. Phase 3 studies study long-term effectiveness and safety in larger groups of persons with Parkinson's. Phase 2 and 3 studies usually have strict inclusion and exclusion criteria, such that persons who may have many other health problems or are on too many medications may be excluded. Phase 4 studies are usually "open label" (which means there is no placebo) and are done after the drug has gained approval by the FDA, to better assess how it performs in the "real world." Phase 4 studies are very important, because they can assess the usefulness and safety of the new drug among the kinds of patients who were excluded in Phases 2 and 3.

Where Can I Learn More?

Whether the research study in which you wish to participate is observational or interventional, make sure you understand all the details before you make up your mind to participate. Inquire about your alternatives, and always ask about the risks and effort involved. You may get more information about clinical trials in Parkinson disease from your health care provider, local academic institutions, the organizations listed in Chapter 13, and the following sources:

- National Institutes of Health: www.clinicaltrials.gov
- Food and Drug Administration: http://www.fda.gov/Science Research/SpecialTopics/RunningClinicalTrials/ucm118862. htm
- PDtrials: www.pdtrials.org

Chapter 12

The Care Partner

Many people do not like being called a "caregiver." That's because they may not provide hands-on care or they don't like a label that suggests some degree of disconnection from their loved one. Some prefer the term "care partner," recognizing that coping with Parkinson disease requires a true partnership. We will use these terms interchangeably throughout this chapter, but we prefer "care partner." No matter what term is used, it is important to acknowledge that both lives are affected by the diagnosis, after which things are never quite the same. Once someone is diagnosed with Parkinson's, a new era has begun for both that person and his or her spouse, partner, or significant other.

Even though a care partner may have recognized changes in the loved one for some time, the official diagnosis of Parkinson's often comes as something of a shock. A common reaction is feeling overwhelmed. How can the doctor know for sure? Shouldn't tests be done? (There are no definitive lab or imaging tests for Parkinson disease.) Should we get a second opinion? (In many cases, that's a good idea.) As medical evaluations and care proceed, it's often helpful for care partners to accompany their loved ones to learn about Parkinson disease.

Care partners are also involved in seeking out information and doing initial research into the diagnosis. Seeking appropriate educational literature through credible organizations and Web sites can be helpful, though it may be best not to bombard your loved one with every detail you learn about Parkinson disease. She or he is probably even more overwhelmed than you are with the implications of a chronic neurologic condition. An informed care partner can be helpful to the loved one by providing reassurance that Parkinson disease is highly "livable," progresses slowly in most patients, and does not appreciably shorten life expectancy.

Discuss together how you will share the news of the diagnosis with friends and family members. If you have children living at home, choose a level of information and an approach that is age appropriate. Learning about or visiting a support group is helpful for some people, but it is important to do your homework and find a group that's a good match for your situation. Recently diagnosed people (and their care partners) may be overwhelmed by support groups made up primarily of individuals who have lived with Parkinson's for a long time. What's more, a recently diagnosed person's concerns will probably not be addressed in the most appropriate manner in such a group.

Be prepared for an initial onslaught of "free advice." Friends and adult children are notorious for suggesting miracle cures they've heard about, herbal supplements, or the latest article they've just read online about Parkinson disease. Be polite, but talk to your physician before proceeding with any of their recommendations.

The care partner will need to recognize that Parkinson disease causes slowness of movement and feelings of fatigue. Patience and a good sense of when help is needed are often required from the care partner. Avoid the tendency to do everything for the person with the disease. Most people prefer to be independent and may resent attempts to provide assistance. Care partners are often helpful simply by being flexible, recognizing that Parkinson disease symptoms may result in changed schedules and plans. Knowing that stress exacerbates symptoms can help care partners understand that asking someone to hurry or rush usually makes the situation even worse.

Worry or concern over a loved one's diagnosis of Parkinson disease is normal. In early stages of Parkinson's, there may be little disruption to the daily routine. It is often not necessary to make major life changes. If changes or accommodations become necessary, it is important to recognize that care partners still need to fulfill their own needs to maintain their health and wellness. Try to keep connections with relatives and friends who nurture your spirit, and continue to make time to do things you enjoy.

The rate of symptom progression in Parkinson disease varies considerably from one person to another. Care partners are urged not to predict problems but to be prepared for changes that are likely to occur over time. As time goes by and symptoms increase, care partners often need to make additional adjustments. In time, fluctuations in the response to levodopa (such as wearing off, on/off phenomena, and dyskinesias) may appear. These fluctuations make it hard to plan activities or predict physical capabilities, since Tuesday may be different than Wednesday. Recognize that these fluctuations are part of Parkinson disease for many people and are not under your loved one's control. It is important to try to be flexible when scheduling activities and events. At the same time, it's important to realize that loss of motivation and even depression can be part of the disease. Sometimes the care partner has to be the "motivator," and it may be challenging to balance encouragement to do more things and keep active with backing off and letting your loved one rest.

People with Parkinson's and their care partners rarely adjust to living with the disease at the same rate. Role conflicts often emerge at this stage of the illness. Renegotiate who can and will do which tasks. (Who should pay the bills? Is it time to hire someone to do the yard work? Is continued driving by the person with Parkinson's beginning to affect the safety of family or others on the road?) These conversations can be difficult, because they reflect the Parkinson's patient's enormous loss of independence, and may result in more responsibility and stress for the care partner. As Parkinson disease progresses, changes in mood and cognition (how the person feels, thinks, and reasons) may become more problematic than motor symptoms. Seek medical guidance when noticing increasing physical symptoms (such as slowness, walking changes, or balance loss) or mental changes affecting safety (such as confusion, hallucinations, paranoia, or dementia). These changes can sometimes be improved with medication adjustment, but they may also signal needs for further adjustment in the daily routine.

Coping with Caregiver Stress and Fatigue

Realistically, caregiver stress is just part of life when caring for a loved one over an extended period. The phrase "caregiver burnout" is sometimes used in the literature but suggests the unfortunate image of a flame extinguished with no hope of relighting the wick. Caregiver distress can be acknowledged, and hopefully managed, only if the person in distress or close, caring observers take notice of the warning signs and are willing to intervene.

Early signs of caregiver fatigue may include the feeling that after several years of increasingly "taking the lead" in your relationship (with no end in sight), life is not turning out the way you'd expected. Voice your concerns and seek assistance as needed. Don't attempt to become a "superhero." Maintain open communication with your loved one and allow time and opportunity to candidly discuss your fears and concerns. Midstage Parkinson disease may also prove an ideal time to share more details about the disease with key friends and family members. If you haven't done so already, make sure crucial planning documents such as a will, a durable power of attorney, and advanced directives are in place (more on this in Chapter 14). Start building your "B Team": people who can help you out in small ways now and familiarize themselves in ways to help if they need to fill in for you in the future, when the need becomes greater.

Signals of increasing caregiver fatigue can take many forms. Fatigue may include growing feelings of isolation. The feeling that "nobody knows or understands what is really going on with us" is always frustrating and is sometimes true. There may be increasing

feelings of anxiety or uncertainty about the future. The care partner's patience may be tested, resulting in outbursts of anger, often
followed by feelings of guilt. Stressed care partners often report
feelings of profound tiredness or exhaustion not relieved by sleep.
Stress-induced physical symptoms (such as recurrent headache,
upset stomach, and other pain) may also occur. Some caregivers
develop problems concentrating and making decisions. They can
experience feelings of depression, bitterness, despair, and hope-
lessness. These warning signals are not to be overlooked. Caregivers
should seek medical evaluation for any physical symptoms and discuss any feelings of stress or depression with a medical provider.
Many care partners benefit from counseling, antidepressants, support from social services, or other interventions designed to help
caregivers cope with increasing fatigue.

Caregivers may wish to acknowledge their stress levels and
fatigue by scheduling a meeting with key friends and family members to candidly discuss what's happening in their lives. Have the
courage to share feelings of isolation, disappointment that friends
have stopped coming to visit, or frustration that family members
are not supportive in the ways you need. Make a short list of *specific*
tasks that would help you take better care of your loved one and
get some much-needed respite. For example, a caregiver could ask
a friend, "Could you come on Tuesdays to take Frank to the barber
or out to lunch?" Be honest if lack of funds is a constant worry; perhaps someone in your circle is able to help with medication costs for
one month or pick up groceries for you once a week. Ask for one or
two volunteers to be "on call" for you during particularly bad days.

If symptoms reach advanced stages and the person with
Parkinson's requires even more care and support, it often becomes
difficult to separate yourself from your role as a caregiver. It is vital
to establish a pattern of taking care of your own physical and mental health needs as well as those of the person with Parkinson's.
Don't put off scheduling a mammogram or neglect a morning walk
because you feel too busy or preoccupied meeting a loved one's

needs. Martyrdom is overrated as a coping mechanism! (If you failed to establish yourself as a co-priority early on, it's never too late to start.)

Private time and relaxation are basic human needs. Make an effort to schedule time away from caregiving responsibilities on a regular basis. Consider drafting a written caregiving plan that specifies that you get, say, one hour per day and one day per week to yourself. To continue giving effectively to the other person, it is essential for long-term caregivers to restore their own energy and "recharge their batteries" on a regular basis. This may even involve something as simple as turning off the cell phone and checking into a nearby hotel. Call on the people who have prepared and trained to serve as your backup team. This is not "selfish." If you become ill or suffer severe burnout, who would possibly be there in the same way for your loved one?

Accept assistance when it is offered, but be mindful of potential caregiver burnout even in your local helpers. For instance, an adult daughter living nearby with a job and children at home may feel as overwhelmed as you do. Be frank with long-distance family members in regard to how they might help. For example, suggest they come and fill in for that long weekend, pay for dental work not covered by insurance, or cover the prescription copay that's become out of financial reach. Family members and friends can also help by phoning every week at an expected time or just sending a card every month; such small gestures can provide amazing comfort in the midst of great distress.

Home care services can offer assistance with caregiving tasks such as bathing and dressing and with other personal needs. If you can afford it, consider paying someone to clean the house and perform household maintenance. Some home care services are covered by insurance, but many require adequate private funds for payment. A social worker or geriatric case manager can help you access available home care services in your community and offer guidance regarding fees and services provided.

Ask the Experts: What Can I Do to Keep Up with the Demands of Being a Care Partner?

One care partner compared her experiences to running a marathon. It's "long and sustained, sometimes tiring, at times feeling never ending, though ultimately a gratifying experience." Both care partners and marathoners need to follow some of the same basic rules to be successful:

- **Train and prepare.** Take time to learn about Parkinson disease and what to expect if symptoms progress. Seek a care partner support group or other venue where you can share your thoughts and feelings with others with similar experiences. Ask questions during medical appointments, and seek referrals to social services, counseling, and other support as needed.
- **Replenish energy along the route.** While time away is important for needed respite, don't underestimate the power of even a short break in the daily routine. A brief walk, a phone conversation with a friend, or just a cup of tea and a favorite TV program can help restore perspective and energy.
- **Protect the body to avoid injury.** Make sure you receive proper instruction in how to best help your loved one. Learn about use of good body mechanics and techniques to safely help your loved one out of chair or off the floor after a fall or to transport a walker or wheelchair in your car. Seek referral to a physical therapist who can instruct you in these matters and so reduce the risk of your being injured.
- **Rest before and after "the race."** Schedule breaks into your day and make sure you are getting enough sleep. Consider arranging overnight assistance a few times each week if you are not receiving adequate rest. Use of the services of adult

(Continued)

(*Continued*)

> day programs or volunteer respite programs may allow you time for daytime sleep.
>
> - **Sometimes walk part of the way.** *No one can do it all, including family caregivers. Recognize that despite your best efforts, some days do not go as planned. Consider ways to simplify the daily routine, and try to reduce any tendency for perfectionism. Keep a few frozen dinners stashed for emergency use, learn to say no to outside requests from others, or make use of delivery services to cut down your daily to-do list.*

Planning for the Future

Be proactive as you consider future plans. These questions are worth discussing with family members and others:

- What will we do if my loved one becomes ill and requires greater levels of care?
- What will we do if I become ill or am no longer able to provide care to my loved one?
- What will we do if neither of us is able to remain in our current situation?

If you are concerned about needing a different place to live for you, your loved one, or both of you, investigate *in advance* the need for and availability of assisted-living and skilled nursing facilities. It may also be helpful to familiarize yourself with palliative (comfort) care options such as hospice, so that if and when the need arises, you will know where to turn.

Take a friend, relative, or geriatric care manager with you to visit a few places and get an idea of the available choices. This is easier than waiting until a hospital stay and discharge necessitates finding a place on short notice. A list of appropriate questions when reviewing facilities may include the following:

- What is the "look" and "feel" as you walk in? Would you be proud for friends and relatives to visit you here?
- How far is the available unit from the dining area? Is everything on one level?
- Are there appealing views or outside spaces?
- Do things seem clean and in good repair?
- Is there a laundry facility for residents?
- What is the level of noise and chaos in the common areas?
- Do a majority of residents have dementia?
- Are you comfortable talking with the marketing director and other staff you meet? How long has the chief administrator held that job? Is a registered nurse available or on call 24/7?
- Do you feel pressure to "decide today" and sign move-in commitment forms? Is there an option to "try before you buy" by staying in a guest room and taking multiple meals in the facility to see if it is a good match for your needs and preferences?
- What do residents say about the food service and dining room staff? Are serving hours flexible? Can the cook accommodate special requests, such as eggs cooked to order? If you are unable to come to the dining room, what is the charge for a tray brought to your room?
- In addition to the basic monthly charge, how much are fees for services such as help with bathing and dressing and medication assistance? Who determines what services you actually need? Can additional services be added to your monthly bill without your prior permission?
- Are hairstyling services available on premises? What is the cost for a haircut, style, manicure, and so on?

- What days are transportation services available? Is there help to get on and off the van and handle packages? Do theses services cover the area where your doctors' offices are?
- In the event of a medical emergency, can you be taken to the hospital of your choice?
- Does the facility have rooms available for people on Medicaid-funded programs, so that you can remain there if your personal funds are spent? What percentage of residents pay out of their own pocket?

If you are a care partner who is an adult child, friend, or other relative, you may consider moving the person with Parkinson disease into your home. Be realistic and consider all options. Ongoing caregiving can bring out the best and the worst of many situations. Your freedom to come and go on short notice may be sacrificed, and caregiving may take time and attention away from other family members, who may act out in unanticipated ways. While children in your home may need to be quieter as a result of having an older relative in the home, older children and teens sometimes become kinder, more thoughtful family members. You may be surprised to find out that friends or other family members can become critical or offer unwelcome advice once you have taken in the person with Parkinson disease. Even though the person you care for may be grateful for your help, be prepared for times he or she appears unpleasant or resentful of the need for constant care. Despite the burden of caregiving, the relationship between you and your care recipient often becomes stronger over time.

A Caregiver's Story: Marilyn

Even though she's married, 73-year-old Marilyn does pretty much everything around the house these days.

"I cut the grass, grocery shop, cook, clean, wash, iron, shovel the snow, take the dog to the vet, take him [her husband, Jim] to the doctor, pick up all the prescriptions, and I make the dental appointments," she says. "Sometimes," Marilyn adds, "I feel like I'm being pulled in one hundred different directions."

Marilyn's husband was diagnosed with Parkinson's 10 years ago. Jim is in his mid-70s now. The disease wasn't bad at first: he had a tremor on one side of his body and had trouble remembering the plots of movies. But over the years, things have slowly become more difficult for Jim—and Marilyn. When he gets dressed, he often misses a button on his shirt and a belt loop on his pants. Because of tremor, he also has trouble combing the back of his hair and shaving his face. He can do it—it's just that he misses spots. When his nose drips, he doesn't notice. So Marilyn has to help him, remind him, prod him.

"I feel more and more overwhelmed," she says. "I'm overwhelmed physically, financially, and emotionally."

Lots of caregivers feel like Marilyn. Taking care of a loved one while taking care of yourself and a house is a big, big job. It's also a job that requires more time than most paid jobs. Here are some of the strategies Marilyn uses to cope:

- **Attend support group meetings.** Marilyn attends a caregivers group that meets every other Monday at a local senior center. The other group members provide tips and share stories. "Listening to the stories helps me know what to look for in the future," Marilyn says. "It's been a great help."
- **Exercise regularly.** In the summer, Marilyn works in the flower garden, tending to her hostas and ferns. Because gardening reduces the stress in her life, Marilyn calls the flower garden her "stress garden." In the winter, she walks on the treadmill in her living room.
- **Make time for friends.** Jim is well enough to go fishing with his buddies and—with the help of family—be on his own occasionally. So Marilyn schedules regular breakfasts and lunches

with friends from high school. Since they've known each other for more than five decades, she feels like she can tell them anything.

- **Make necessary changes in the house.** Marilyn and Jim love each other, but they sleep in twin beds now, because Jim gets up frequently in the middle of the night to go to the bathroom. The noise wakes up Marilyn, but the twin beds allow her to get a good night's sleep. They've also added a railing to Jim's bed to make it easier for him to get out of bed.
- **Ask for help when you need it.** Marilyn's adult children live nearby, so sometimes she asks for help with big outdoor chores. They've got busy lives, but somehow they find the time to lend a hand. Although she takes pride in doing all the housework herself, she hired window washers for the first time in more than 50 years because she just can't do everything.
- **Plan for the future.** Marilyn and Jim have their wills and power of attorney documents completed (see Chapter 14).
- **Don't do everything.** Jim needs lots of help, but he's not helpless. One time when he asked Marilyn to look up a phone number for him, she encouraged him to find it himself. Although he ultimately wasn't able to find it without help, she felt the nudge encouraged him to be independent in areas where he is capable.
- **Enjoy the little things.** At about the time Jim was diagnosed with Parkinson disease, the couple bought a miniature schnauzer. The dog has been a great companion for Jim, following him around the house and joining him on the recliner at night. And when Jim goes to bed, the dog curls up with Marilyn.

A Caregiver's Story: Rich

Another caregiver, Rich, offers these thoughts: "Parkinson's is a disease that you must take a day at a time and respond to whatever challenges that particular day brings. An extra phone call or trip to the doctor may not provide any relief, because the problem of the day may simply be the general progression of the disease. On the other hand, since the disease causes changes in the patient, a conversation with the doctor may result in a modification in medication or a change in some recommended therapy that may help return the quality of life closer to normal.

"As each day brings its own challenges, there is nothing better for the patient than to know his family and caregivers are ready, willing, and able to help in any way that is necessary. Our family always tried to be there for my father and to help with his special requests when my mother was not able to do so. We always encouraged him to get out of the house and even simply run errands with my mother just to give him a change of scenery and get his mind off the constant worry about the progression of the disease."

Chapter 13

Community Involvement, Advocacy, and Resources

Parkinson disease isn't just about medication, coping, and loss. Many people find that becoming active in a support group or advocacy organization adds a sense of belonging and purpose to their life. That is just as true for people with Parkinson disease, their care partners, and families.

Attending support group meetings to share common problems and worries is helpful for many people. There are a number of support groups, both online and in person. Some groups are focused on the recently diagnosed, care partners, or people with young-onset Parkinson disease. Before attending a meeting, it's a good idea to find out more about a group's audience and goals to see if it's a good fit for you.

There are also opportunities for involvement in Parkinson's research studies. These studies come in a variety of forms: surveys, medication trials, interviews, and other types of participation. It is important to ask questions about the study's design, along with any potential benefits or risks, before deciding to participate. Your physician may be aware of research studies in your area, or you can investigate a number of ongoing studies at www.pdtrials.org or by calling the Parkinson's Disease Foundation at 800–457–6676. (Chapter 11 has more information on research.)

Although there are a variety of ways to become involved in Parkinson-related activities, each individual must decide on her or his own level of interest and comfort in doing so. Some people find it upsetting to be involved in activities where other people are in more advanced stages of the disease. Some are not comfortable sharing their thoughts and feelings in a group setting. There is no right or wrong decision on getting involved. The decision is yours. Some people with Parkinson disease choose to become involved through advocacy, fund-raising, or volunteerism. Many people feel that a sense of involvement contributes to their overall quality of life. To find out more, contact one of these national organizations:

American Parkinson Disease Association
800–223–2732
www.apdaparkinson.org

Michael J. Fox Foundation for Parkinson's Research
800–708–7644
www.michaeljfox.org

National Parkinson Foundation
800–327–4545
www.parkinson.org

The Parkinson Alliance
800–579–8440
www.parkinsonalliance.org

Parkinson's Disease Foundation
800–457–6676
www.pdf.org

Parkinson's Action Network
800–850–4726
www.parkinsonsaction.org

Many cities and states are also home to independent Parkinson groups. In addition, most U.S. states are home to local affiliates of the American Parkinson Disease Association or the National Parkinson Foundation, two of the groups listed above. See their Web sites or call those organizations for information on local chapters.

A Passion for Advocacy

Jackie Hunt Christensen has always been a bit wonky. After college, she worked as a public policy advocate for Greenpeace and then shifted her emphasis to agricultural trade issues. "I've always worked for action-oriented organizations," she says. "It's a natural thing for me."

At age 32, Jackie suspected something wasn't quite right with her physically. Two years later she was diagnosed with Parkinson disease. Today, Jackie is 46 years old and a fierce advocate for people living with the disease. She has served on the board of directors of the Parkinson Association of Minnesota, has coordinated state efforts for the Parkinson's Action Network, and recently organized a one-day Parkinson conference at a local university.

"It's in my blood," she says. "I feel like if I'm not doing something actively to make life better, the disease wins. I'm not ready to concede that yet."

Jackie has also written two books: *The First Year: Parkinson's Disease: An Essential Guide for the Newly Diagnosed* and *Life with a Battery-Operated Brain: A Patient's Guide to Deep Brain Stimulation Surgery for Parkinson's Disease.* Not everybody has to be as involved as Jackie to have an impact on the lives of others. In fact, Jackie wishes lots of people would take small steps to help the public better understand Parkinson disease.

"In my definition of advocacy, anyone who doesn't let the disease keep them imprisoned in their own home is an advocate," she says. "Simply by going outside or going to church and being willing to answer questions, you are an advocate." Jackie believes that people need to be educated about an issue before you can get them to do something. So educating someone in your neighborhood, a member of your church, synagogue, or mosque, or anyone else about the disease makes you an advocate. Most people have an extremely limited view of what Parkinson disease is. By asking questions, they are showing a desire to learn more. Jackie hopes more people living with Parkinson's will help educate folks.

"I feel strongly that the actual patient voice needs to be adequately represented," she says. Jackie recommends first talking to others one-on-one about the disease and then becoming comfortable talking to small groups at a place of worship or local civic organization.

"Ease into it," she says. As for Jackie, she's also going to keep advocating for people with the disease and their families.

"I can't imagine not being able to do this."

A Passion for the Arts and Helping Others

Bright colors illuminate the paintings of Sheila Moriarty. Sometimes the colors are magnificent, as in the sweeps of orange, green, and yellow that fill a rendering of flowers. In other works, the colors are subtle. In one painting of a church on a winter day, the eye is drawn to snow clinging to a barren tree. But soon it drifts to a bluish green sky that suggests a wish for spring.

Sheila, 76, didn't begin painting until she received a diagnosis of Parkinson disease. She paints with watercolors because it's less time-consuming than other forms of painting.

"I only work in watercolors because it's fast," she says. "I fear I don't have much time before my medication wears off." She adds, "I paint for the love of it."

But Sheila's not the only one who loves the paintings. Her paintings have been purchased at art fairs, church sales, and silent auctions. The Parkinson's Disease Foundation has featured her watercolors on its Web site. A Scottish Parkinson's organization has adopted one of her paintings as its logo. And she often donates paintings to fund-raisers for Parkinson-related causes. Sheila donates her paintings to these causes because she wants to make a difference in the lives of people.

"It gives me a thrill, because it's like I'm part of the research team," she says. "I can help."

Sheila isn't the only one who feels this way. Many people with Parkinson disease or family members of someone with the disease feel empowered by giving back to the community. They do it in lots of ways.

Kevin Burkart raises money for Parkinson groups by jumping out of airplanes. Kevin's father has the disease. So in 2008, Kevin promised to make 100 skydives in a single day—but only if people donated money to local and national Parkinson groups. The event raised more than $40,000. In 2010, Kevin parachuted from an airplane 200 times in one day. That fund-raiser, called "200 Perfect Jumps," generated more than $60,000 for Parkinson-related causes.

Of course, there are plenty of more conventional ways to raise money for Parkinson advocacy and research. Many state organizations sponsor walkathons, bike rides, golf tournaments, bowlathons, charity runs, tea parties, auctions, bake sales, and other community events.

Find Out More

Support groups and advocacy groups aren't the only places to learn about Parkinson disease. There are many free online sources and free pamphlets you can access. When searching for information on the Internet, it's important to look for sites, magazines, workbooks, and pamphlets published by trusted organizations. Here are some more resources:

Neurology Now
800–422–2681
www.neurologynow.com
(A free bimonthly magazine published by the American Academy of Neurology that includes many articles on Parkinson disease and related therapies)

We Move
www.wemove.org
(A Web site with information for patients and their families presented by the Movement Disorder Society, an international association of movement disorders experts)

Parkinson's Hope Digest
www.parkinsons.hopedigest.com

PDWebcast: Parkinson's Science: Innovations and New Perspectives
Parkinson's Disease Foundation
www.pdf.org/en/webcast

National Sleep Foundation: Parkinson's Disease
703–243–1697
www.sleepfoundation.org

Understanding Parkinson's Plus Syndromes and Atypical Parkinsonism
Parkinson's Disease Foundation
800–457–6676
www.pdf.org/en/factsheets

Medications, Fourth Edition
By David Hougton, MD, and co-authors
National Parkinson Foundation
800–327–4545
www.parkinson.org

Activities of Daily Living: Practical Pointers for Parkinson Disease
By Heather Cianci, PT, MS., GCS, and co-authors
National Parkinson Foundation
800–327–4545
www.parkinson.org

American Speech-Language-Hearing Association (ASHA)
800–638–8255
www.asha.org

Be Independent: A Guide for People with Parkinson Disease
By Nancy A. Finn, PhD, OTR/L, and co-authors
American Parkinson Disease Association
800–223–2732
www.apdaparkinson.org

Directory of Certified Specialists in Physical Therapy
American Physical Therapy Association
800–999–2782
www.apta.org

The Importance of Physical Therapy and Exercises for People with PD
By David Lehman, PhD, and Mark A. Hirsch, PhD
Parkinson's Disease Foundation
800–457–6676
www.pdf.org/en/factsheets

Lee Silverman Voice Treatment (LSVT)
888–438–5788
info@lsvtglobal.com
www.lsvtglobal.com

The Science and Practice of "Speaking LOUD"
By Lorraine Ramig, PhD, CCC-SLP, and Cynthia Fox, PhD, CCC-SLP
Parkinson's Disease Foundation
800–457–6676
www.pdf.org/en/factsheets

Good Nutrition News (fact sheet)
American Dietetic Foundation
800–877–1600
sales@eatright.org

Ask the Parkinson Dietician (online forum)
National Parkinson Foundation
forum.parkinson.org

Be Active: A Suggested Exercise Program for People with Parkinson's Disease
By Terry Ellis, PT, PhD, NCS, and co-authors
American Parkinson Disease Association
800-223-2732
www.apdaparkinson.org

Eldercare Locator Service
Area Agency on Aging
800-677-1116
www.eldercare.gov

Job Accommodation Network
Office of Disability and Employment Policy
U.S. Department of Labor
800-526-7234
www.askjan.org

BenefitsCheckup
www.benefitscheckup.org
Melvin Weinstein Parkinson's Foundation
757-313-9729
www.mwpf.org
(This organization helps low-income Parkinson's patients)

Family Caregiver Alliance
800-445-8106
www.caregiver.org

National Family Caregiver Association
800-896-3650
www.thefamilycaregiver.org

Visiting Nurse Association of America
202-384-1420
www.vnaa.org

Chapter 14

Planning for Your Future: Managing Your Personal Affairs

Murray Sagsveen, JD, and Laurie Hanson, JD

We all know in theory that we should plan for unexpected family emergencies such as the diagnosis of a chronic illness. Day-to-day matters often allow us to push this kind of planning to the bottom of our "to do" list, however. Planning for emergencies by necessity involves difficult family discussions that we might prefer to avoid. However, addressing difficult family decisions before an emergency arises is usually far easier than coping with them during an emergency.

To illustrate, consider the following example:

John visited his aging mother, Bertha, and they discussed the importance of an advance directive and a power of attorney. Bertha insisted that she did not want the family to take any unusual life-prolonging measures if something were to happen so that she could not make decisions for herself. She asked that John handle her finances if she were to become unable to do so. After this conversation, John made an appointment with his mother's attorney, and after several more discussions among the three of them, Bertha decided to sign an advance directive and a durable power of attorney. A month later, Bertha had a severe stroke that did in fact leave her unable to communicate.

If John had not started this discussion with his mother about an advance directive and power of attorney, Bertha's other children might never have learned about her end-of-life wishes. Had John and Bertha not taken the time to have an advance directive and power of attorney discussed, drafted, and signed, John would not have been able to handle even routine financial matters for his mother after her stroke.

This chapter explains the importance of planning for the future *and* provides useful information to assist you and your family with these details. You will learn ways to ensure that your affairs are managed as you want them to be managed—even if you are no longer able to communicate or make decisions yourself.

You will learn about the following:

- **Informal arrangements with friends or family**
- **Formal arrangements with or without court involvement**
  - **To manage your financial affairs, such as powers of attorney, trusts, and conservatorships**
  - **To manage your health care through health care directives, living wills, POLST, DNR/DNI/DNHs, or guardianships**
  - **To ensure that your post-death wishes are followed regarding your property and the disposition of your body**

Your Emergency Notebook

A first step in planning for emergencies is assembling and maintaining key health, financial, and other information in one place, so that family members and caregivers can access the information if you are suddenly unable to communicate with them. Many organizations have developed planning guides that are free for members. But you can also create your own "emergency notebook" with a three-ring binder and a set of divider tabs. Organize your emergency notebook as follows, with tabs separating documents into the following sections:

1. Emergency contact information
   - Spouse, partner, or significant other
   - Children
   - Siblings
   - Parents
2. Financial and legal contact information
   - Estate attorney
   - Accountant
   - Investment advisor
3. Medical information
   - Medication (recent, past, and present)
   - Contact information for both primary care and specialist physicians
   - Immunization records
   - Significant medical, dental, and eye care details (including the physicians' names and locations of medical records)
   - Allergies
   - Significant family medical history
4. Financial information
   - Bank accounts
   - Insurance policies
   - Retirement plans
   - Stocks and bonds
   - Recurring bills (for example: utilities, insurance, mortgage payments)
   - Real and personal property
   - Loans (receivable and payable)
   - Financial powers of attorney
   - Taxes (location of past tax returns and information for current tax year)
   - Safe deposit box

5. End-of-life information
   - Will and any accompanying statement concerning final arrangements for personal property
   - Advance directive
   - Organ donor information
   - Funeral and burial guidance
6. Location of key items
   - Important documents (for example: passports, military records, deeds, marriage license, Social Security numbers, titles to vehicles)
   - Photos
   - Jewelry
7. Passwords and electronic media (Passwords are vital, and given that they frequently change, don't forget to update your emergency notebook, even if by hand.)
   - Home and office computers
   - Software programs
   - Financial and medical Web sites
   - Facebook and similar pages (consider, for instance, how you want these handled after your death)

Of course, an emergency notebook is not helpful if family members cannot find or access it. When discussing the contents of your emergency notebook with family members, be sure to explain where the notebook is located.

Informal and Formal Arrangements

A second step in emergency planning is to make arrangements for events that may be anticipated or unanticipated. Depending on the circumstance, the arrangements made will be either informal or formal.

Informal Care Arrangements

Informal arrangements are temporary and can usually be made with family, friends, and neighbors. For example, if you have surgery scheduled and know that you will be unable to perform normal household chores while you are recuperating (an anticipated event), you may want to line up family members or friends to assist with your medication, grocery shopping, cooking, transportation to medical appointments, or housekeeping. You may also want them to help with financial matters, such as writing out checks, filling out tax returns, and balancing the checkbook. Such informal arrangements are very common and, in fact, make up the majority of assistance to people who are temporarily or permanently living with disabilities.

Entrusting private financial or medical information to family members or friends, however, may have unintended negative consequences. It may result in uncomfortable situations that may even have financially or medically harmful consequences. In such cases, formal arrangements are preferable. Formal arrangements may include legal safeguards regarding supervision and record-keeping, or review by an outside party to minimize the risk of exploitation by an informal caregiver. Similarly, formal arrangements may also be made to protect the caregiver, who may later be questioned regarding legitimate reimbursement for services.

Even when informal arrangements work well, the day may come when more formal arrangements are needed.

Formal Financial Management Services

When planning for the future, it is important to know what financial management services are available for your individual needs. These services are listed next, starting from the least to the most formal.

Automatic Banking and Direct Deposit

Modern banking technology, such as automatic bill payment and direct deposit, can help you with your finances. At a minimum, Social Security payments and pension income should be set up so they are directly deposited. Utilities and insurance payments should also be set up to be withdrawn automatically from your account. Doing so can prevent you from unintentionally discontinuing your health insurance or from having your electricity shut off. It is wise to have one "working" bank account, such as a checking account, into which income is deposited and from which monthly bills are paid.

To arrange for Social Security checks to be deposited directly to a bank account, you may call Social Security at 1-800-772-1213 and ask for a direct deposit form or sign up on the Social Security Direct Deposit page online at http://www.ssa.gov/deposit/. A bank can also provide you with this form. Beginning in 2013, all Social Security recipients will be required to have checks directly deposited.

Multiple-Name Bank Accounts

Adding a name to a bank account is an easy and effective way to allow a trusted relative or friend to provide informal help. By having access to the account, that person can help sign checks, pay bills, or transfer money between your accounts. That person can also have access to bank records to monitor electronic deposits, ensure that all bills are paid on time, and review monthly statements to ensure that nothing is amiss in all your accounts.

Several types of multiple-name bank accounts are available, each with different rules. Any type of account—for example, savings, checking, and certificates of deposit—may be held in more than one name. Such accounts are easy to set up just by visiting the bank. However, great care must be taken to select the appropriate type of account (as explained next) for your situation and to assure that you have selected a trustworthy person to help you.

The following types of multiple-name accounts are commonly available:

Joint Account

In a joint account, any person whose name is on the account is considered a co-owner. Each named person can make deposits and withdrawals without the other person's knowledge or consent. There are a few facts about joint accounts to keep in mind:

- The other person could withdraw all of your money without consequence or legal recourse.
- The other person's creditors could tie up the funds in the account (with a lien or attachment) until proof of your ownership of the funds is provided.
- A person's name cannot be taken off the account without that person's written approval.
- In a joint account, when one owner dies, the survivor automatically owns the account without going through probate court. This can be a benefit because the funds are immediately available to pay urgent expenses, such as funeral costs. It can also have negative consequences if the joint account holder is not your intended beneficiary.

Authorized Signer Account

An authorized signer account, or a convenience account, allows another individual to make deposits and withdrawals to your account and sign your checks. The other signer's creditors cannot tie up your account. However, as with joint accounts, there is still the risk that the other authorized signer could withdraw all your money from your account. Unlike a joint account, the account does not belong to the other authorized signer upon your death; rather, funds in this account belong to your estate—or to a named beneficiary (see later). The authority of the other signer ends with your death, so the other authorized signer will not be able to use the funds after your death.

Payable on Death Accounts and Beneficiary Designations

All checking, savings, investment, and retirement accounts allow you to designate to whom your account will be distributed at your death. Sometimes these accounts are called payable on death (POD) accounts. Both the beneficiary designation and the POD account allow for planning after your death, but these designations do not affect ownership during your life. The named beneficiary cannot make withdrawals or sign checks, so it is a useful way to bypass probate to give money to loved ones after your death.

Naming a Representative Payee

A representative payee is an individual or organization appointed by the U.S. Social Security Administration, the U.S. Office of Personnel Management, the U.S. Department of Veterans Affairs, or the U.S. Railroad Retirement Board who may be charged with receiving your income, using that income to pay your current expenses, saving for your future needs, and maintaining proper records. The Social Security Administration has a Representative Payee Program with rules and regulations to protect the beneficiary of the income. Learn more about the Representative Payee Program at http://www.socialsecurity. gov/payee. To have the authority to manage your Social Security or Supplemental Security Income benefit, a person or organization must be appointed by the Social Security Administration. A power of attorney or note from you is not good enough. Having a representative appointed provides oversight that may give you assurance that your bills and finances will be properly handled. Many professional fiduciaries and organizations serve as representative payees.

Family Caregiving Contracts

Individuals are often uncomfortable with the idea of paying family members or friends for caregiving arrangements. But changes

in the Medicaid asset transfer rules over the past 15 years, as w--
as the reality that caregivers must sometimes give up their day jobs
in order to provide the necessary level of care, have made personal
care contracts an attractive option, both to make sure that the level
of care is met and that children (or other relatives or friends) do not
have to sacrifice their own financial well-being while providing care
to their parents.

Personal care contracts must, as a general rule, be in writing and
state the kind and extent of services that are necessary, within reasonable terms. Because personal services contracts involve payment
for services, income paid to a family caregiver through such a contract is subject to payroll and income taxes, and caregivers should
consult an accountant to ensure that the income is reported properly. Tax credits are not available for parent caregiving unless the
parent is the child's legal dependent.

Durable Power of Attorney

A power of attorney is an extremely important planning tool.
It allows you to appoint someone to manage all of your financial
affairs if you are unable to manage them yourself. If no power of
attorney exists and it is necessary to liquidate or transfer assets or
enter into real estate transactions (including those of a spouse),
it may be necessary to go to court to establish a conservatorship
before these matters can be acted on. Establishing a conservatorship can be costly and time-consuming. Thus, everyone should have
a power of attorney.

Power of Attorney Defined

A **power of attorney** is a written document in which you (as the
"principal") appoint another person (the "attorney-in-fact") to handle your property or finances. The power of attorney can be effective

for all purposes or for a limited purpose (for example, appointing another person to sign a deed for the sale of your home when you are unavailable). A power of attorney becomes ineffective if the principal becomes incapacitated or dies.

Durable Power of Attorney Defined

A "durable" power of attorney continues to be valid even after the principal becomes incapacitated. A durable power of attorney document must specifically state that it is "durable" and must contain specific language, such as "This power of attorney shall continue to be effective if I become incapacitated or incompetent." Generally, if the purpose of a power of attorney is to make sure that someone can manage your finances when you cannot, the power of attorney should be durable.

Care Must Be Taken in Choosing an Attorney-in-Fact

Powers of attorney are not supervised by courts, so they can be abused if the wrong person is appointed attorney-in-fact. While the attorney-in-fact is required by law to act in the best interest of the principal, it is difficult to get your money back if the person you have appointed handles your affairs unwisely. Therefore, you must choose someone you trust implicitly—a person who will *always* act in your best interests.

Creating a Power of Attorney

While forms are available free on the Internet, it is best to consult an experienced attorney to create a power of attorney. Too many times, individuals sign documents they have printed off the Internet only to discover later that the documents are invalid or do not serve their purposes. This can be a very costly error, because it may be necessary to have a court appoint a conservator to do what could have been accomplished easily with a validly executed power of attorney.

Safeguards to Protect You

You may trust a friend or family member to be your attorney-in-fact and feel confident that no safeguards are necessary. However, another option is to hire a professional fiduciary, such as a bank trust department, to ensure that your finances are handled the way you want. Either way, consider including the following safeguards in a power of attorney:

- Require that the attorney-in-fact provide an annual or monthly accounting to you, your lawyer, an independent accountant, or a trusted family member to review.
- Name two attorneys-in-fact on the document and specify that they must act jointly (for example, both attorneys-in-fact must agree and both must sign checks).
- Require your appointed attorney-in-fact to obtain a surety bond to cover the value of your property if the attorney-in-fact mishandles your funds.
- Appoint a successor in case the attorney-in-fact dies, becomes incompetent, or simply chooses not to act on your behalf.

Cancelling or Ending a Power of Attorney

A power of attorney can be canceled or revoked at any time. Each state has specific requirements for revoking a power of attorney. Your revocation should be sent to the attorney-in-fact and to any person or institution with whom the attorney-in-fact has done business on your behalf.

Remember, a power of attorney becomes invalid if the principal become incompetent or dies. However, a *durable* power of attorney continues if the principal becomes incompetent and can be revoked only by a guardian or conservator, if one has been appointed. A durable power of attorney terminates when the principal dies.

Trusts

A trust is a legal arrangement in which a person or a financial institution owns and manages assets for your benefit. The parties to a trust are the person setting up the trust (the "grantor"), the person or organization administering the trust (the "trustee"), and the person for whom the trust is established (the "beneficiary"). Often the grantor and the beneficiary are the same person.

An agreement, called a trust instrument, between the grantor and the trustee explains the trustee's authority. A trust can be created by the terms of the grantor's will (a **testamentary trust**) or during the grantor's lifetime (a **living trust**, also called an inter vivos trust). A living trust is the type of trust used to manage assets during a time of incapacity. Some trusts are court supervised, and some are not.

Trusts are not for everyone. A living trust is generally not appropriate for modest estates because the costs and disadvantages, including the time and logistics involved in administering them, outweigh the benefits. As with any planning tool, it is important to review each option for managing estates to determine the strategies that best fit your situation. In other words, one size does not fit all.

Basic Living Trust Defined

You may create a living trust during your lifetime by transferring ownership and control of your assets to the trust.

A trust can be revocable or irrevocable:

- As long as you are competent, you may change, revoke, or terminate a **revocable trust** at any time during your lifetime. A revocable trust is normally used for property management purposes. After you die, the revocable trust becomes irrevocable.

- A revocable living trust is often used as a planning tool because it allows a trustee to manage your property for your benefit during life and can also provide for distribution or ongoing management after your incapacity or death. Most commonly, in a living trust you would be both your own trustee and beneficiary. As such, your Social Security number would be used when establishing trust accounts or doing trust business. You would manage your property as if the property were in your name. A trust agreement would also include your directions should you become incompetent or die. If you have a medical condition that could result in your being unable to manage your affairs, a revocable living trust may be the right choice.
- An **irrevocable trust** cannot be changed or terminated after it has been established. It is a separate taxable entity, requiring its own tax identification number. Tax considerations may be a factor in deciding whether to make a trust revocable or irrevocable, particularly when a substantial amount of property is involved.

Care Must Be Taken in Choosing a Trustee

A trustee has as much, if not more, responsibility as an attorney-in-fact in a power of attorney. Great care must be taken in choosing your trustee. In most revocable living trusts, you would serve as trustee as long as you are able to do so. Should you become incapacitated, the "successor trustee" would take over and be responsible for management of all trust assets during your life and for distribution of those assets to the beneficiaries upon your death. Being a trustee is a huge responsibility and should not be taken lightly. While a family member or other individual could be named trustee if you are sure that person is trustworthy and capable of acting in this capacity, a fair amount of expertise is needed to handle the paperwork, tax returns, and property management tasks that may be involved. In most cities, professional trustees are available for hire, and many banking institutions have trust departments. Going over options with an attorney before naming a trustee is always wise.

Creating a Living Trust

A revocable living trust is established with the execution of a trust agreement. In this document, you would name the beneficiary (usually yourself during life), state how the property should be managed if you become disabled, and direct how the property should be distributed at your death. A living trust is much like a will in this way, and so many states require specific formalities in signing a trust to ensure that you are not being coerced or unduly influenced by someone in executing the trust. Trusts should be drawn up by an attorney familiar with drafting them.

To receive the advantages of the revocable trust, all assets must be placed in the trust or the trust must be named beneficiary.

Important Tip

Be on guard against anyone who uses high-pressure tactics to sell a living trust package. Do not deal with anyone who demands a signature right away or requires money before you have time to do additional research. Some companies only want to sell their prepackaged plans and do not assist clients in putting assets into the trust. These trusts can cause problems that will be expensive to fix.

A Revocable Trust Cannot Be Used to Avoid Paying Nursing Home Costs

A revocable trust is considered an available resource under Medicaid laws and is not a way to avoid spending savings on nursing home care. The federal and state Medicaid laws are very complicated and subject to change at any time. Do not try to use a trust without getting competent legal advice.

Trusts for Protecting Assets While Dependent on Medicaid

People living with chronic conditions may ultimately require assistance with activities of daily living (ADLs), such as bathing, transferring, ambulation, eating, toileting, and basic hygiene and grooming. This type of assistance is known as custodial care. Individuals may receive this care at home, or they may need to move to an assisted living facility or a nursing home. No matter where these services are received, they are very expensive. Medicare does not cover the cost of custodial care. Long-term care insurance policies may cover these types of costs. However, it is difficult to obtain long-term care insurance after you are diagnosed with a significant medical condition. When long-term care insurance is not available, private funds must be used to pay for the cost of care. Once private funds are depleted, many individuals turn to Medicaid to pay for these services.

Medicaid eligibility rules are complex and vary depending on (among other things) the state in which you reside, whether you are married or single, the types of services you need, and your age. As a very general rule, however, you may keep a car and your home (as long as you are living in it) and about $3,000. Be aware that this amount varies from state to state. The point is, you can have only limited assets outside of your home and car. There are three types of trusts available that, if properly established and administered, allow a person with a disability to retain more than $3,000 and still be eligible for Medicaid to pay for the cost of care. These three trusts are a first-party special needs trust, a third-party special needs trust, and a pooled trust. The funds in any of these three trusts may be used to purchase goods and/or services that "supplement and do not supplant" government benefits. In other words, funds in the trust may be used for goods and/or services that benefit the individual and do not replace the government benefits the individual receives. For instance, funds may be used to pay for a companion dog, nonconventional treatments, massage, companion services, a home, rent, travel, or clothing. Funds may not be used to pay for medical services covered by Medicaid. Because you can have only $3,000 to be eligible for Medicaid to pay the cost of custodial care, having a special needs trust can make a significant difference in your life. Sometimes a special needs trust can make the difference between living at home or in a nursing home.

First-Party Special Needs Trust

A first-party special needs trust is a way for an individual to place his or her own money into a trust and remain eligible for Medicaid. It is called a "first-party" special needs trust because the individual's assets are used to fund the trust. Assets in a first-party special needs trust remain exempt if:

- The trust is established by a parent, grandparent, guardian, or court and is:
  - For the sole benefit of the person with the disability as certified by the Social Security Administration
  - For a person who is under the age of 65
  - Using the person's assets—this includes any assets a person may be awarded as a result of a personal injury lawsuit
- The trust is irrevocable by the beneficiary and may only be changed by the trustee if the change is necessary to comply

with a new law or decision governing first-party special needs
trusts.

- The trust has a provision that at the death of the person with
the disability, any remaining trust assets must be distributed first to the state as repayment for any Medicaid that
has been received.

Third-Party Special Needs Trust

A third-party special needs trust is a way for a third party to give
money to a person with a disability in a way that does not jeopardize
the individual's eligibility for public benefits. For instance, if a parent or grandparent or best friend wants to leave money to a person
with a disability, or if friends want to throw a fundraiser, a third-
party special needs trust is used. Sometimes third-party trusts are
set up while the grantor is alive; other times they are set up in wills.
Assets or funds belonging to the person with the disability must
never be placed in the trust. There is no payback to the Medicaid
Agency. Rather, the grantor may state who will receive any funds
remaining in trust at the beneficiary's death. Laws regarding the
supplemental needs trusts vary from state to state, and a lawyer
should be consulted in each state.

Pooled Trust

A pooled trust is a type of special needs trust, and for all intents
and purposes it is administered like a first-party special needs
trust. However, a pooled trust must be established and managed by a nonprofit corporation. A separate subaccount must be
maintained for each beneficiary of the trust, but, for purposes
of investment and management, the trust pools the accounts.
Each subaccount must be established solely for the benefit of
individuals who are disabled as defined by the Social Security
Administration. The subaccount may be set up by the parent,

grandparent, or legal guardian of the individual, the individual him or herself, or by a court. To the extent that amounts remaining in the subaccount at the beneficiary's death are not retained by the pooled trust, the trust must pay such remaining amounts to the state in an amount equal to the total amount of Medicaid paid on behalf of the individual.

Health Care Directives

A **health care directive**, often called an advance directive, is a written document in which you appoint someone (a health care agent) to make health care decisions in the event you are unable to make them yourself.

A health care directive is now recognized as a combination of two earlier documents: the living will (a document that provides specific guidance to physicians, nurses, and caregivers about medical treatment) and a durable power of attorney for health care (a document that authorizes another person to make health care decisions when you are unable to do so).

Why Create a Health Care Directive?

You have the right to make decisions about your health care, including the right to refuse treatment, authorize treatment, and access information in your medical records. In a health care directive, you can authorize a trusted loved one, relative, or caregiver (the designated health care agent) to make necessary health care decisions according to your wishes if you are unable to do so yourself.

What Must a Health Care Directive Include?

Health care directives are governed by state law, and most state laws have several statutory requirements. Most important, a health care directive must be written by a competent person, and be dated, signed, and witnessed or notarized.

Who Can Be a Health Care Agent?

Your health care agent may be any individual 18 years of age or older who is not your health care provider or an employee of your health care provider. You should choose someone who you know well and trust to make decisions according to your wishes. It is very important to discuss your wishes in detail with a prospective health care agent before you finalize your decision. Make sure the person clearly understands your wishes *and* appreciates the responsibilities involved. You should also name a successor (backup) health care agent in case the primary health care agent is unable to act when decisions must be made.

What Is Included in the Health Care Directive?

In your health care directive, you may:

- Appoint one or more agents or alternative agents and include instructions for how decisions should be made and whether named agents must act together or may act independently
- State a preferred nursing home in the event such care is necessary
- State which medical records the health care agent can access
- State that the health care agent is the "personal representative" under the federal Health Insurance Portability and Accountability Act (HIPAA) and has the authority to access your medical records
- State whether the health care agent shall be guardian or conservator if a petition is filed

- State whether your eyes, tissues, or organs should be donated on your death
- Make a declaration regarding intrusive mental health treatment or a statement that the health care agent is authorized to give consent for such treatment
- State specific instructions if you are female and pregnant
- Give instructions regarding artificially administered nutrition or hydration
- State under what circumstances the health care directive will become effective
- State any other instructions regarding care, including how religious beliefs may affect health care delivery
- Provide instructions about being placed on a ventilator, receiving resuscitation, or other aggressive measures if there is minimal to no chance that you will recover
- State what will happen with your body at death (body identification/burial/cremation)

When Do the Health Care Agent's Responsibilities Begin?

Generally, the health care agent may make decisions for you when your physician believes you are unable to make your own decisions.

What Are the Duties of the Health Care Agent?

The health care agent is obligated to make informed, good-faith health care decisions from your point of view. The health care agent should follow your guidance in the health care directive and should seek legal help if the medical providers will not comply with his or her requests.

Can the Health Care Directive Be Cancelled or Revoked?

You may cancel or revoke the health care directive in whole or in part by:

- Destroying the document
- Executing a written and dated statement explaining what part of the health care directive you want to revoke
- Verbally expressing the intent to revoke it in the presence of witnesses
- Executing a new health care directive

Where Should the Health Care Directive Be Kept?

The health care directive must be readily available in an emergency. It should be kept with your personal papers in a safe place—such as your emergency notebook—(not in a safe deposit box unless someone else is also a signer on the box). You should give signed copies to family members, close friends, your health care agent, your backup health care agent, and your doctors so that they can include it in your medical records.

What Is the Uniform Anatomical Gift Act?

The Uniform Anatomical Gift Act allows you to donate your entire body, organs, tissues, or eyes for research or transplantation. If you do not make the gift, close relatives, a guardian, a conservator, or a health care agent may make an anatomical gift at the time of death—unless it is documented that you refused to donate organs while alive. Verification of intent to make an anatomical gift may be indicated on your driver's license.

Is a DNR/DNI/DNH the Same as a Health Care Directive?

The acronym DNR/DNI/DNH means "Do not resuscitate/do not intubate/do not hospitalize." This is a request by a patient to his or her physician to limit the scope of emergency medical care. The request is signed by the patient or the patient's proxy, and it must be ordered by a physician. It will be followed by emergency medical personnel if presented to them at the time of the emergency. You should have a health care directive as well, because the DNR/DNI/DNH is limited only to decisions regarding end of life and resuscitation or intubation and does not deal with all other myriad issues that may arise at the end of one's life.

What Is POLST and Is It the Same as a Health Care Directive?

POLST stands for Physician Orders for Life-Sustaining Treatment. It is an initiative that began in Oregon in 1991 in recognition that patient wishes for life-sustaining treatments were not being honored despite the availability of advance directives. POLST has endorsed programs in about 14 states and programs under development in many other states. It is a signed medical order that can be used by emergency medical technicians and other health care professionals during an emergency. The form is more specific than an advance directive and is signed by the patient's provider, making it a medical order. The physician must meet with the patient to go over the form and learn treatment options available for the specific disease or serious illness the patient has. Like the DNR/DNI/DNH order, POLST is not meant to take the place of an advance directive or the appointment of the agent.

Where Can I Obtain Health Care Directive Forms?

An attorney who specializes in eldercare law or has experience with health care directives can prepare a directive that is tailored to your needs.

In addition, suitable forms may be downloaded from reputable Web sites, such as the following:

- Aging with Dignity: http://www.agingwithdignity.org/five-wishes.php
- American Bar Association: http://www.abanet.org/publiced/practical/directive_whatis.html
- National Hospice and Palliative Care Organization: http://caringinfo.org/i4a/pages/index.cfm?pageid = 3289
- U.S. Living Wills Registry: http://liv-will1.uslivingwillregistry.com/forms.html
- The Departments of Health in individual states

Guardianship and Conservatorship

Guardianships and conservatorships are relationships between two people created by the court to protect people who cannot handle their own financial or personal affairs. Definitions vary from state to state. Most generally, a **guardian** is appointed for the purpose of managing the personal affairs of a person who has become incapacitated (called a ward), including making personal decisions and meeting needs for medical care, nutrition, clothing, shelter, or safety. A **conservator** is appointed for a person (called a protected person) for the purpose of managing finances, assets, and income when it has been shown that the person has impaired ability and/or judgment. If a person needs both a guardian and a conservator, one person may be appointed by the court to fill both of those roles.

A Guardianship or Conservatorship Is Required When No Plan Is in Place

A guardianship or conservatorship is necessary when a person becomes unable to handle finances or live safely without help and no previous arrangements have been made. The decision to obtain a guardianship or conservatorship should not be made lightly because it takes away the person's most basic right: to make decisions about his or her own health and welfare. The court will appoint a guardian or conservator who will handle all of the person's affairs, including perhaps where he or she will live.

The court will appoint a guardian or conservator only if a less restrictive alternative is not available for managing the personal and financial affairs of the person. It is likely that no guardianship or conservatorship will be necessary if a health care directive and a power of attorney have been put into place.

> It is likely that neither a guardianship nor conservatorship will be necessary if a health care directive and a power of attorney have been put into place.

Establishment of a Guardianship or Conservatorship

While practices may vary state by state, generally a guardianship or conservatorship is established by filing a petition with the probate court in the county where the person resides. Anyone can ask the court to appoint a guardian or conservator for a person who needs help. The potential ward or protected person must be given advance notice of the hearing and has the right to be represented by an attorney at any court proceeding, even if he or she cannot pay for the attorney. In this case, the court will order the county to pay these costs. The person requesting a guardianship or conservatorship must prove through clear and convincing evidence that such an order is necessary. This could be difficult if the proposed ward or protected person does not want a guardianship or conservatorship established.

Your Will

A **will** is a set of written instructions about how to dispose of your assets upon death. Assets are either described as probate assets or nonprobate assets. Probate assets are those assets whose ownership a court must rule on following the owner's death. Nonprobate assets are assets that will automatically transfer to another person at death such as those with joint tenancy or beneficiary designations or assets that have been placed in a trust. Probate court is the court charged with determining ownership either by administering a legal will or by state law when no legal will exists.

Not Everyone Needs a Will—But It Is a Good Idea

If property is held in such a way that it will pass through beneficiary designations or joint ownership, then a will is not technically necessary. However, a will is necessary if a person wants personal property, such as jewelry, paintings, and family heirlooms, distributed in a certain way. Tax or private family matters may exist that make it wise to use a will and probate court to administer an estate. Finally, even if there seems to be no reason for a will, having one is the best way to ensure that an individual's wishes will be followed.

GLOSSARY

Acetylcholine: One of the neurotransmitters.

Adrenaline: A hormone produced by the adrenal glands (small glands sitting on top of the kidneys). This chemical is used by some nerve cells of the autonomic nervous system to communicate with organs such as the heart, the gut, the skin, and the pupil of the eye.

Agoraphobia: A condition in which a person becomes very anxious or panicky in crowded situations or just on being outside their home.

Akathisia: An inability to sit still, caused by an "ants in the pants" feeling. This is different from restless legs in that it is not under voluntary control

Akinesia: Inability to move or initiate voluntary movement.

Antioxidants: Chemicals or nutrients that scavenge free radicals, the toxic by-products of natural chemical processes that take place inside normal or diseased cells.

Antipsychotic drugs: Medications used to control psychotic symptoms (for example, hallucinations, delusions, and paranoia).

Apathy: Loss of interest, motivation, or emotional response.

Apraxia: Inability of the brain to plan, initiate, and execute certain tasks or even simple voluntary movements.

Atypical parkinsonian syndrome: A condition that resembles Parkinson's but is caused by a different disease. The term is used when there is insufficient evidence to make a more precise diagnosis such as multiple system atrophy or progressive supranuclear palsy.

Autonomic nervous system: The part of the nervous system that controls automatic or involuntary functions of the body. In simple terms, these are functions that a person doesn't have to think about, such as heartbeat, sweating, and the movements of our stomach and intestines.

Basal ganglia: Clumps of nerve cells deep inside the brain whose job is to work out the details of most voluntary actions. For example, when a movement is initiated, it is the job of the basal ganglia to ensure that the movement is accurate, smooth, and performed with adequate speed.

Benign tremulous parkinsonism: A form of Parkinson disease in which there is a lot of tremor but relatively little rigidity or bradykinesia.

Blood–brain barrier: A complex system of cells in the brain that control the entry and exit of chemicals and nutrients into and out of the brain.

Bradykinesia: Slowness of movement.

Bradyphrenia: Slowness of thinking processes.

Camptocormia: Crookedness of the trunk.

Carbidopa: A medication that blocks the breakdown of levodopa outside the brain, thereby maximizing the amount of levodopa that ends up in the brain and cutting back some of its side effects, such as nausea.

Carbidopa/levodopa: A pill that contains both of these medications.

CBD: See *Corticobasal degeneration.*

Chorea: Involuntary and uncontrollable dancelike movements.

Cognition: The combined functions of the brain that have to do with the thinking processes.

Cognitive dysfunction: A malfunction of the thinking processes of the brain.

COMT inhibitors: A group of anti-Parkinson drugs that work by blocking the breakdown of levodopa, thereby prolonging its effectiveness.

Conservator: An individual appointed to be responsible for managing finances, assets, and income of an individual who is incapacitated (a protected person).

Corticobasal degeneration: A neurodegenerative disease that shares some features with Parkinson disease and may sometimes look like Parkinson disease.

DBS: See *Deep-brain stimulation.*

Deep brain stimulation: A brain surgery that introduces a wire into the brain through which the activity of certain areas of the brain can be regulated to restore normal function.

Dementia: Cognitive dysfunction that is sufficient to cause significant impairment in one's day-to-day activities and is not due to a reversible cause. The most well-known dementia is Alzheimer disease, but dementia can be caused by many diseases, including Parkinson disease.

Dementia with Lewy bodies: A neurodegenerative disease that combines features of Parkinson disease with early dementia.

Diplopia: Double vision.

Disease modifying: A term used to describe medications that may alter the course of disease progression (ideally by slowing it down).

DLB: See *Dementia with Lewy bodies.*

DNA: The material of which genes are composed.

Dopamine: One of the neurotransmitters.

Dopamine agonist: A drug that exerts its action by stimulating dopamine receptors.

Dopamine receptors: Proteins through which dopamine exerts its actions.

Dopaminergic: Using a dopamine-related mechanism.

Dopaminergic neurons: Nerve cells that produce and use dopamine to communicate.

Duodenum: The first part of the small intestine, immediately downstream from the stomach.

Dys-: A prefix used to mean difficult or abnormal.

Dysarthria: Slurred speech.

Dysautonomia: Dysfunction of the autonomic nervous system.

Dysexecutive syndrome: A type of cognitive dysfunction that affects executive functions of the brain, such as planning and organizing one's actions, taking initiative, solving problems, managing different tasks simultaneously, and performing complex tasks that require multiple choreographed steps.

Dyskinesia: Abnormal, involuntary movements as a side effect of medications.

Dysphagia: Difficulty with swallowing.

Dysphonia: Difficulty with producing a strong or clear voice.

Dystonia: Abnormal, involuntary movement that results from the simultaneous contraction of muscle that have opposing actions. Dystonic movements are slow, cramped, and usually follow a repeating pattern. Alternatively, dystonia is a disease characterized predominantly by dystonic movements.

Emotional lability: Inability to control emotional outbursts, such as crying or laughing with very little provocation.

Exercise physiologist: A professional who specializes in the use of therapeutic exercise.

Executive function: The function of the brain that has to do with planning our actions, making decisions, directing our attention, stopping us from doing things we consider inappropriate, detecting and correcting mistakes, and making choices.

Feeding tube: A thin, flexible tube inserted into the stomach or the duodenum, usually through the nose and the esophagus, for the purpose of administering nutrition and medications in people who have lost their ability to swallow temporarily.

Free radicals: By-products of normal chemical processes that occur inside cells. Free radicals can cause oxidation, permanently damaging normal components inside cells, a process that has been considered central to the aging process and cell death. Normal cells have mechanisms to prevent this damage, and some nutritional supplements and vitamins can help. These "good chemicals" are called antioxidants.

Freezing: A symptom in Parkinson disease, but also in other diseases, in which one's feet feel glued to the ground.

Frequency: In the context of Parkinson disease, this usually means having to urinate frequently.

Gastrostomy: A procedure in which a tube is inserted into the stomach or the duodenum through the skin of the abdomen, to provide a way to administer nutrients and medications to people who have lost their ability to swallow.

Gene: A portion of a cell's DNA that contains the blueprint for the cell to build a specific protein.

Genome: The full list of all the genes in a species (for example, humans, dogs, rats, or monkeys).

Globus pallidus: A structure in the basal ganglia, often used as a target for deep-brain stimulation surgery in Parkinson's.

Guardian: A person appointed for the purpose of managing the personal affairs of an individual who is incapacitated (a ward). A guardian is responsible for making personal decisions for the ward and for meeting the ward's needs for medical care, nutrition, clothing, shelter, or safety.

Hallucination: A perception of something that does not exist (for example, seeing dead people or hearing music that's not there).

Health care directive: A written document, often also referred to as an advance directive, in which an individual appoints someone (a health care agent) to make health care decisions in the event that the individual cannot make them independently and to give instructions regarding health care.

Hereditary: Transmitted through the genes.

Hoehn and Yahr scale: A staging system for Parkinson disease.

Hyper-: A prefix used to mean increased, excessive, or enhanced.

Hypersomnolence: Excessive sleepiness.

Hypo-: A prefix used to mean decreased, deficient, or suppressed.

Hypokinesia: Decreased mobility or movement.

Illusion: Misinterpretation of sensory stimuli. For example, a person might look at a bush and misinterpret it as a person crouching.

Insomnia: Sleeplessness.

Irrevocable trust: A trust that may not be changed or terminated after it has been established. It is a separate taxable entity, requiring its own tax identification number.

L-dopa: See *Levodopa*,

Lee Silverman Voice Treatment: A specialized speech therapy program to improve voice in Parkinson patients.

Levodopa: A drug that is the raw material for making dopamine.

Lewy body: A collection of damaged proteins inside nerve cells affected by Parkinson disease.

Living trust: A trust created during the grantor's lifetime. Also called an inter vivos trust.

LSVT: See *Lee Silverman Voice Treatment*.

Magnetic resonance imaging: A scan of the brain using a high-power magnetic field.

MAO-B inhibitors: A class of anti-Parkinson medications that block one of the enzymes that breaks down dopamine.

Micrographia: A symptom of Parkinson disease, where handwriting becomes small and difficult to read.

Mitochondria: Components of cells that specialize at extracting energy from oxygen.

Motor symptoms: Symptoms having to do with movement and mobility.

Movement disorders specialist: A neurologist who specializes in Parkinson disease and other diseases that affect mobility and movement, such as dystonia and chorea.

MPTP: A chemical that kills dopamine neurons and can cause a Parkinson-like illness in people and monkeys.

MRI: See *Magnetic resonance imaging.*

Multiple systems atrophy: A neurodegenerative disease that combines features of Parkinson's with early and prominent dysautonomia or ataxia (a motor dysfunction similar to being drunk).

Myoclonus: Sudden, jerky, fast, and unpredictable involuntary movements.

Neurodegenerative: Related to premature death of neurons that does not result from a specific cause such as injury, chemicals, tumors, or strokes.

Neurogenic bladder: Urinary bladder dysfunction that results from a disease of the nervous system.

Neurologist: A medical specialist who specializes in diseases of the nervous system.

Neuron: A nerve cell.

Neuroprotective: Protecting nerve cells from disease-related damage, or a drug that has this effect.

Neuropsychologist: A psychologist who specializes in assessing cognition.

Neurosurgeon: A surgeon who specializes in surgery of the brain and of nervous system structures in general.

Neurotoxin: A poison that affects nerve cells.

Neurotransmitter: 1. A naturally occurring substance produced by nerve cells and used to communicate with other nerve cells or organs. Dopamine, acetylcholine, norepinephrine, serotonin, and glutamate are some of the most important neurotransmitters in the brain. 2. The "battery pack" that generates the electrical stimulation in deep-brain stimulation.

Nocturia: The condition of having to urinate frequently at night.

Norepinephrine: One of the neurotransmitters.

Normal-pressure hydrocephalus: A condition where the abnormal accumulation of excess spinal fluid in the cavities of the brain (the ventricles) produces symptoms similar to those of Parkinson disease.

Nutritionist: A health care professional who specializes in proper nutrition.

Occupational therapist: A health care professional who helps people improve their abilities to perform their daily activities, from getting in and out of bed to bathing, showering, writing, cooking, using utensils, improving hand dexterity, and so on.

On/off phenomenon: The occurrence of mostly unpredictable spells during which anti-Parkinson drugs lose their effectiveness.

Orthostatic hypotension (or postural hypotension): A significant drop in one's blood pressure upon standing up that may lead to light-headedness or even fainting.

Pallidotomy: A type of DBS surgery, where the stimulating electrode is placed in the globus pallidus

Pallidum: See *Globus pallidus.*

Parkin: A protein in neurons; mutations in the gene that is responsible for producing this protein causes genetic form of Parkinson's.

Parkinson disease: A neurodegenerative disease characterized by the loss of dopamine neurons in the substantia nigra.

Parkinson disease dementia: Dementia that may occur in the advanced stages of Parkinson disease.

Parkinsonism: A constellation of symptoms similar to those of Parkinson disease. Many diseases and some drugs can cause parkinsonism without causing Parkinson disease.

Pathology: Abnormal changes that happen in tissues, organs, and cells as a result of illness or injury. Also, the medical specialty that deals with investigating such changes.

PD: Parkinson disease.

PDD: See *Parkinson disease dementia.*

Percutaneous endoscopic gastrostomy: A procedure to provide a way to administer nutrients and medications to people who have lost the ability to swallow. A tube is inserted into the stomach or the duodenum through the skin of the abdomen with the aid of a flexible "telescope" inserted in the stomach through the mouth and the esophagus.

Peripheral neuropathy (or polyneuropathy): A condition in which nerves are damaged that convey messages from the spinal cord to the muscles and other organs and that also bring information back to the spinal cord and brain (including sensations such as touch, pain, and temperature).

Physical therapist: A health care professional who helps patients with mobility, balance, or musculoskeletal problems through specific therapies and exercises and through other non-medication treatments, such as ultrasound, heat application, and special equipment.

Placebo: A "dummy" pill that contains no active drug but looks and tastes the same as one that does.

Postural instability: A decline in one's ability to remain standing without losing their balance.

Power of attorney: A written document in which an individual (the principal), appoints another person (the attorney-in-fact) to handle property or finances.

Progressive supranuclear palsy: A neurodegenerative disease that can look very much like Parkinson's, especially in its early stages.

Proteasome: A component of cells that recycles old or damaged proteins.

PSP: See *progressive supranuclear palsy*

Psychiatrist: A medical specialist who diagnoses and treats diseases that present with emotional and behavioral symptoms, such as depression, anxiety, or schizophrenia.

Psychologist: A health care professional who diagnoses and treats psychiatric disorders through non-medication therapies.

Psychosis: A disorder in which patients have altered perceptions of reality. Examples include paranoia and schizophrenia.

RBD: See *REM sleep behavior disorder.*

REM sleep behavior disorder: A sleep disorder in which affected persons "act out" their dreams.

Restless legs syndrome: A condition in which a person has an uncomfortable sensation in their legs while sitting or reclining. The condition is often relieved by getting up and walking.

Revocable trust: A type of trust normally used for property management purposes. Such a trust may be changed, revoked, or terminated at any time during the lifetime of an individual as long as he or she is competent. After death, a revocable trust becomes irrevocable.

Rigidity: Muscle stiffness.

Sensory symptoms: Abnormal sensations of numbness, tingling, pain, or changes in vision, hearing, taste or smell.

Serotonin: One of the neurotransmitters.

Social worker: A professional who can assist patients with understanding insurance and disability issues, getting help in the community and finding the right living situation (such as assisted living or a nursing home).

Speech pathologist: A health care professional who provides therapies for speech, voice, and swallowing problems.

Stereotaxic surgery: A type of brain surgery where a sophisticated technique is used to place probes or wires in deep parts of the brain with great precision and without extensive cutting through the brain.

Striatum: One of the basal ganglia structures.

Substantia nigra: The basal ganglia structure that contains the dopamine neurons.

Subthalamic nucleus: A structure in the basal ganglia, often used as a target for deep-brain stimulation surgery in Parkinson's.

Synuclein: A protein in found in neurons; mutations in the gene that is responsible for producing this protein cause a genetic form of

Parkinson's. Synuclein is one of the proteins that accumulate in Lewy bodies.

Testamentary trust: A trust created by the terms of the grantor's will.

Thalamotomy: A surgical procedure used to control tremor. It consists of making a controlled small lesion, like a mini-stroke, in a part of the brain called the thalamus, in order to "reset" the circuits in the brain that are responsible for the generation of the tremors.

Thalamus: A cluster of cells in the deep parts of the brain with many "relay" functions, including transmission of motor and sensory signals. It can be seen as the central switchboard of the brain.

Tremor: Involuntary rhythmic shaking of a limb.

Ubiquitin: A protein in found in neurons; ubiquitin is one of the proteins that accumulate in Lewy bodies.

Unified Parkinson's Disease Rating Scale: A scale used to rate the severity of Parkinson's symptoms.

UPDRS: See *Unified Parkinson's Disease Rating Scale*.

Urgency: A sensation that one has to urinate immediately.

Video swallowing assessment: A modified X-ray that assesses the swallowing function.

Wearing off: The loss of anti-Parkinson effect toward the end of the interval between medication doses.

Will: A set of written instructions outlining how an individual wishes to have her or his assets distributed uon death.

ABOUT THE AUTHORS AND CONTRIBUTORS

Sotirios A. Parashos, MD, PhD: Neurology Consultant, Minneapolis Clinic of Neurology; Lead Physician for Clinical Research, Struthers Parkinson's Center, Park Nicollet Methodist Hospital, Golden Valley, Minnesota; Adjunct Associate Professor of Neurology, University of Minnesota.

Rose L. Wichmann, PT: Center Manager and Physical Therapist, Struthers Parkinson's Center, Park Nicollet Methodist Hospital, Golden Valley, Minnesota; Faculty, Allied Team Training Program, National Parkinson Foundation.

Todd Melby: Reporter and Radio Producer, Minneapolis, Minnesota.

Sierra Farris, PAC, MPAS: Neurological Physician Assistant, Deep Brain Stimulation Program, Seattle Swedish Medical Center, Seattle, Washington; Core Faculty, Parkinson's Care Consortium, University of Toledo; Teaching Associate, Department of Neurological Surgery, University of Washington.

Susan Imke FNP, GNP-C: Nurse-Practitioner, Kane Hall Barry Neurology, Bedford, Texas; Advisory Board Member, Parkinson

Alliance; Allied Team Training Program, National Parkinson Foundation; Educational Consultant, American Parkinson Disease Association.

Demetrius M. Maraganore, MD: Ruth Cain Ruggles Chairman, Department of Neurology, and Medical Director, NorthShore Neurological Institute, NorthShore University HealthSystem; Clinical Professor of Neurology, Pritzker School of Medicine, University of Chicago.

Martha A. Nance, MD: Medical Director, Struthers Parkinson's Center, Park Nicollet Methodist Hospital, Golden Valley, Minnesota; Adjunct Professor of Neurology, University of Minnesota.

Murray Sagsveen, JD: Currently the chief operating officer and general counsel of The GOD'S CHILD Project. Previously, he was the general counsel of the American Academy of Neurology, chief executive officer of a state department of health, the general counsel of a state medical association, a partner in a law firm, and a judge advocate and brigadier general in the Army National Guard.

Laurie Hanson, JD: Shareholder with Long, Reher & Hanson, P.A., an elderlaw firm in Minneapolis established to represent individuals and family members who are aging and/or living with disabilities. Ms. Hanson concentrates her practice exclusively in disability planning. Ms. Hanson is a member of the National Academy of Elder Law Attorneys and the Special Needs Alliance, a national professional association of attorneys committed to helping individuals with disabilities, their families, and the professionals who represent them.

About the American Academy of Neurology

The American Academy of Neurology, an association of more than 25,000 neurologists and neuroscience professionals, is dedicated to promoting the highest quality patient-centered neurologic care. A neurologist is a doctor with specialized training in diagnosing, treating, and managing disorders of the brain and nervous system such as Parkinson's disease, brain tumors, Alzheimer's disease, stroke, migraine, multiple sclerosis, and epilepsy.

For more information about the Academy and its resources for people with neurologic disorders, visit *AAN.com*. To sign up for a free subscription to *Neurology Now®*, the Academy's magazine for patients and caregivers, visit *NeurologyNow.com*.

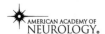

About the American Brain Foundation

The American Brain Foundation, the foundation of the American Academy of Neurology, is one of the largest providers of neurology research grants in the United States. The Foundation supports vital research and education to discover causes, improved treatments, and cures for brain and other nervous system diseases. Learn more at *CureBrainDisease.org*.

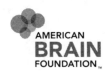

INDEX